Intimate Issues

21 Questions Christian Women Ask About Sex

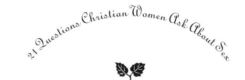

Intimate Issues

CONVERSATIONS WOMAN TO WOMAN

LINDA DILLOW &
LORRAINE PINTUS

WATERBROOK
PRESS

INTIMATE ISSUES
PUBLISHED BY WATERBROOK PRESS
2375 Telstar Drive, Suite 160
Colorado Springs, Colorado 80920
A division of Random House, Inc.

All the stories in the book are true, but names and circumstances have
been changed to protect the identities of the persons involved.

ISBN 1-57856-149-3

Library of Congress Cataloging-in-Publication Data
Dillow, Linda.
    Intimate issues : answers to 21 questions women ask about sex / Linda Dillow
and Lorraine Pintus.—1st ed.
        p.   cm.
    ISBN 1-57856-149-3
    1. Sex—Religious aspects—Christianity—Miscellanea.
2. Christian women—Religious life—Miscellanea.   I. Pintus, Lorraine.
II. Title.
BT708.D54   1999
248.8'43—dc21   98-53167
                                                                          CIP

Printed in the United States of America

2002

15   14   13

To Jody.
Thank you for being my lover
and my best friend for thirty-five years.
Linda

To Peter.
You are my beloved.
Thanks for sharing the journey with me.
Lorraine

Contents

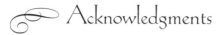 Acknowledgments

A special thanks to:

Liz Heaney, our relentless editor who never let us settle for second best. We thank God for your editing abilities and your friendship.

Rebecca Price and Dan Rich at WaterBrook Press. Thank you for seeing the need for this book. We appreciate your commitment to truth and your willingness to "push the envelope" in creativity.

Our book review committee: Tamara Farrah, Gayle Haggard, Carey Holm, Carole Mayhall, Cindy Smith, Phyllis Stanley, and Mimi Wilson. Your wisdom and insightful comments made this a better book.

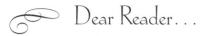 Dear Reader . . .

A preacher was invited to give a talk at a women's health symposium. His wife inquired about his topic, and he was too embarrassed to admit he had been asked to speak about sex. Thinking quickly, he replied, "I'm talking about sailing."

The next day at the grocery store a young woman who had attended the lecture recognized the minister's wife. "That was certainly an excellent talk your husband gave yesterday," she said. "He really has a unique perspective on the subject." Somewhat chagrined, the minister's wife replied, "Funny you should think so. I mean, he's only done it twice. The first time he threw up, and the second time, his hat blew off."[1]

Many people are embarrassed to talk about sex while others blare SEX! from the rooftops. Making public what God intended to be private seems to have become a national pastime. Recently, we saw a television newsmagazine that featured a couple explicitly describing how Viagra had catapulted them into wild ecstasy. We flicked the off button in disgust. Then, a week later, we read a newspaper article about the captain of a South African Airways jumbo jet who had to leave the cockpit to scold two passengers who were openly engaging in sex in the plane's business section.[2]

Everywhere we turn, people are talking about sex. Yet, Christian wives have few places to turn for biblical, frank information from a woman's viewpoint on this sensitive topic. We wrote *Intimate Issues* to provide this much needed perspective.

Before we go any further, let us tell you about ourselves. We are not sex therapists, psychologists, or sociologists. We are students of the Scripture, women who seek God and want to know Him and reveal Him in every aspect of our lives, including our sexual relationships with our husbands. We are both authors and speakers who teach on marriage and the sexual relationship, but also on spiritual-life issues.

In preparation for this book, we asked one thousand women, "If you could have two questions answered about the sexual relationship between a husband and wife, what would they be?" The most frequently asked questions became the chapter titles of this book. We'd like to thank the many women who not only asked the questions, but gave us permission to tell their stories so you might receive wisdom and encouragement. We appreciate their candor, and we've protected them by changing their names.

As part of our research, we read through the Bible from Genesis to Revelation, noting every reference to sexuality. We are concerned that Christian women grow in their sexuality from God's perspective. We wish we could sit down over a cup of coffee or tea and talk about your questions and pray with you over your concerns. Because this is not possible, we have asked God to meet with you as you read this book. And, we've asked Him to help you feel you are not only meeting with Him, but also with two friends who care for you.

We have spent hours in prayer over this book. We wanted to be specific enough to be helpful, but sensitive enough not to offend. God has declared that His gift of sex in marriage is to bring abandoned pleasure and intimate oneness. May this book reveal His heart and may you be motivated and encouraged to grow to become both a godly and sensuous wife.

We are praying for you,

Linda & Lorraine

Linda and Lorraine

For more information about products by these authors
or to learn about Intimate Issues Conferences, visit
www.intimateissues.com.

HOW TO READ THIS BOOK

Intimate Issues can be used

- as a handbook to help you transform your sexual attitudes and enhance your sexual relationship;
- for personal reflection (an application section called "Change My Heart, O God" is included at the end of each chapter);
- as a resource for counseling other women;
- for individual or group Bible study (a twelve-week study is included at the end of the book).

Each chapter is self-contained so that you can turn to a specific question and find the help you need. However, we recommend that you read straight through the book as certain themes build upon one another. In either case, be sure to read chapters 1 and 2, as they contain foundational information.

We have divided the twenty-one questions into three sections. Part 1 contains "Simmering Questions" that are always in the back of our minds. Part 2 covers those "Smoldering Questions" that burn and cause pain, and Part 3 provides wise answers for those "Sizzling Questions" that are so "hot" they need immediate answers. The sealed section at the back of the book holds an Intimate Secret, which offers step-by-step instructions for exciting romance with your spouse. We recommend that you don't read the Intimate Secret until you have worked through the entire book.

We have chosen to include numerous stories from women we've talked with and have quoted both Christian and secular resources. We have only quoted secular sources when they offer help or insight that is not contrary to Scripture. Please understand this does not mean we are recommending the book or magazine, only the portion we have quoted.

part one

Simmering Questions

one

What Does God Think About Sex?

*Y*ou are standing in the grocery store checkout line, wishing the checker would move more quickly, when you get the urge for a piece of gum. As you reach for a pack of Dentyne, the headline from a nearby tabloid shouts:

ORGIES KEEP MY MARRIAGE ALIVE

Next to this, a woman's magazine announces:

SEVEN WAYS TO SEDUCE YOUR MAN

Your eyes scan the magazine racks. Every tabloid and woman's magazine screams a similar message at you. In an attempt to silence them, you look away and study the vegetables in your basket. All you wanted was a piece of gum, but you got more to chew on than you had bargained for! As you contemplate your broccoli, you pray, *God, I know sex orgies are wrong, but what about a wife seducing her husband? Where do I draw the line on sexual acts? What is right? What is wrong? Can I be both godly and sensuous? I wish I knew how I should think about sex and how You, God, think about sex.* I want to feel sexual — I want to love to love my husband & must feel dumb.

If you feel confused when it comes to sex, you are not alone. Most women have not grasped God's view of sex. They are unsure what He thinks because His voice is often lost in the discordant symphony of voices clamoring to be heard. With so many mixed messages, it's no wonder many are confused.

CONFLICTING VOICES CAN CAUSE CONFUSION

If we listened to the *Victorian voices,* we'd be confused.

> "Don't talk about *it;* stay under the covers with the lights off."

> "Do *it* only in the missionary position."

> "*It* is only for men."

> "Chin up, honey. Just endure *it.*"

If we listened to the *voices of sexual pioneers,* we'd be confused. Psychologists Sigmund Freud, Henry Havelock Ellis, Alfred Kinsey, William Masters, and Virginia Johnson called for women to come out from under their "Victorian covers" and be sexual creatures. While their words contained positive components, their tone often offended our sensibilities.

> Here is how your body works. Plug this prescription into your body computer and BINGO, it will orgasm. It's every woman's right, make your "personal computer" do its thing.

If we listened to the *voices of certain church fathers,* we'd be confused.

> Augustine allowed that sex is good but passion and desire are sin. "For he who is intemperate in marriage, what is he but the adulterer of his own wife."[1]

> Thomas Aquinas thought as long as sex was not enjoyed,[2] marriage was acceptable for those unable to accept the requirements of monastic existence.

> Martin Luther had these words to say: "Intercourse is never without sin; but God excuses it by his grace because the estate of marriage is his work."[3]

Sex without passion or enjoyment? Intercourse a sin? With such a heritage no wonder Christian women are confused.

If we listened to the *voices of mothers,* we'd be confused. Of course, some mothers gave wise advice, but others sent negative messages:

"Only 'those kinds' of girls enjoy sex."

"Sex is a man's thing. You just endure it."

And the least helpful response: S I L E N C E.

If we listened to the *voices of some older married women,* we'd be confused. Many equated sex with duty and often complained:

"Wait until you've been married twenty years, it gets old."

"After two years of marriage, the excitement vanishes. You'll see."

"Give him his sex so you can have your children."

If we listened to the *voice of the media,* we'd really be confused.

Sex always just happens naturally.

The woman is always instantly passionate, instantly ready. She never needs love, encouragement, or foreplay. Her sexual glands activate at the unbuttoning of a shirt.

Both the man and the woman know everything, do everything just right, and are instant perfect lovers.

Tiredness vanishes with one passionate look.

Neither the man nor the woman ever has morning breath. The woman wakes up, makeup in place, the man's hair neatly combed.

Does any of this sound familiar? All of these voices have influenced the way we view our sexuality. God's thoughts about His gift of sex have been so distorted that many women don't know what to believe. Some wonder if something is wrong with them.

"In movies making love looks so simple. Couples fall into bed in fits of passion. They catch their breath, and then go at it again. I feel like something is wrong with me. I need foreplay, time to be aroused sexually. I can't see myself spending two days in bed. I guess I'm just not very sensuous."

"Sometimes when we make love, I have something on my mind about the children, our home, the gardening, and it's hard for me to get into lovemaking. What's wrong with me?"

"I grew up confused about sex. It was obvious my parents avoided one another. Now that I'm married, the magazines at the newsstand say there is something wrong with me if I don't have this compulsion to dress up like Jane and swing around the room with my Tarzan. Whom do I listen to? No matter what I do, it's wrong."

There *is* something wrong, but not with these wives. What's wrong are the voices. On the one hand they whisper that sex is evil, and on the other hand they yell, "Do it!" Anytime, anywhere with anyone. Multiple positions, multiple orgasms, multiple multiples!

This is not what God intended. It's time to silence the voices who cry in the darkness and listen instead to the One Voice who whispers the truth in the light. Do you hear Him? God is calling you, pleading with you to hear His voice. He who made us has much to say about sex—He invented the idea. Let's open our ears. Open our eyes. Open our hearts.

God's voice—His Word—tells us why He created sex.

GOD'S VOICE DECLARES:
"I GAVE THE GIFT OF SEX THAT YOU MIGHT CREATE LIFE"

God formed Adam from the dust of the earth. Then He fashioned Eve from Adam's rib. He could have continued creating man and woman in this way or chosen from a multitude of other options available to Him. But in His perfect wisdom, God designed sexual intercourse as the best plan for man and woman to create a new life. Beginning in Genesis, we are commanded to "be fruitful and multiply, and fill the earth" (1:28). This may be the only commandment given by God that His people have consistently applied. The gift of sex gives us the unspeakable privilege of creating a child from our love. How incredibly creative our God is!

Some have wondered if God instructed Adam and Eve: "This is what you do to make a baby . . ." We don't think so. God exquisitely crafted the man and woman's bodies so that they would mold and fit together. Can you imagine Adam and Eve's amazement and wonder when they discovered this? And their glorious ecstasy when they held their baby in their arms, a creation of their love?

GOD'S VOICE DECLARES:
"I GAVE THE GIFT OF SEX FOR INTIMATE ONENESS"

"A man shall leave his father and his mother, and shall cleave to his wife; and they shall become one flesh" (Genesis 2:24). Isn't this an incredible thought? Two separate beings become so bonded, so connected, so woven together in body, soul, and spirit that God sees them as one being rather than two.

The apostle Paul quotes this verse and expounds upon its meaning. He describes the one flesh between husband and wife as a great mystery. A mystery is usually something secret or hidden, but Paul makes the mysterious plain. God's Word says our sexual oneness is an earthly picture of the spiritual oneness Christ is to have with His church (Ephesians 5:31-32).

In light of this, how can anyone say God thought sex was wrong or dirty when He, the almighty Creator of the universe, said our physical oneness is to be a picture of the spiritual oneness He wants to have with us? It's as if God is saying, "Through your lovemaking, I've given you a visual picture so that when you experience the beauty of physical intimacy, you will have a glimmer, an earthly idea, of all I desire for you spiritually, a sweet union of your spirit with mine." Such glorious oneness is almost beyond comprehension.

GOD'S VOICE DECLARES:
"I GAVE THE GIFT OF SEX FOR KNOWLEDGE"

In Genesis 4:1 (NKJV) we read, "Now Adam knew [had sexual intercourse with] Eve his wife, and she conceived and bore Cain." The Hebrew word for "sexual intercourse" is the word "to know." Through God's gift of sex, a husband and wife receive an intimate knowing of one another that they have with no one else. This knowledge brings a depth to their relationship. Mike Mason says it beautifully in *The Mystery of Marriage.*

> For in touching a person of the opposite sex in the most secret place of his or her body, with one's own most private part, there is something that reaches beyond touch, that gets behind flesh itself to the place where it connects with spirit, to the place where incarnation happens.[4]

GOD'S VOICE DECLARES: "I GAVE THE GIFT OF SEX FOR PLEASURE"

Would you believe Scripture talks more about the pleasures of sex than it does about "being fruitful" and "being one"? God devoted an entire book of the Bible, the Song of Solomon, to the subject of sexual pleasure in marriage. Many other passages also speak of the joys of married love. Listen to God's voice:

> Drink from your own well, my son—be faithful and true to your wife.
> . . . Let your manhood be a blessing; rejoice in the wife of your youth.
> Let her charms and tender embrace satisfy you. Let her love alone fill
> you with delight. (Proverbs 5:15,18-19, TLB)

The first part of this verse draws a beautiful parallel between thirst being quenched by drinks of cool, fresh water and a couple's sexual thirst being satisfied by exciting, pleasurable lovemaking. The second part of the verse describes the emotion a couple experiences when they embrace. Our favorite paraphrase of this passage reads:

> Let your love and your sexual embrace with your wife intoxicate you
> continually with delight. Always enjoy the ecstasy of her love.[5]

It would be difficult to find stronger words than *intoxicate* and *ecstasy.* These are God's words, this is His voice saying to you, "Enjoy your husband, give to him, receive from him. Delight yourself in the erotic feelings of sexual love."

GOD'S VOICE DECLARES:
"I GAVE THE GIFT OF SEX AS A DEFENSE AGAINST TEMPTATION"

God's gift of sexuality can be used as a powerful force for good or for evil. To make certain His gift was used for good—to create a child, to give unique knowledge, intimate oneness, pleasure, and comfort—God wrapped His gift within the bonds of the marriage vows. Proverbs warns young men about the temptations of sexual lust and encourages them to "Drink water from your own cistern, and fresh water from your own well" (5:15). The following passage makes it clear that sex in marriage is a deterrent to temptation:

> But because of immoralities, let each man have his own wife, and let each woman have her own husband. . . . Stop depriving one another, except by agreement for a time that you may devote yourselves to prayer, and come together again lest Satan tempt you because of your lack of self-control. (1 Corinthians 7:2,5)

GOD'S VOICE DECLARES:
"I GAVE THE GIFT OF SEX FOR COMFORT"

Part of God's plan for sex is to impart comfort. Listen to this account in 2 Samuel where David and Bathsheba's son has died. While grieving "David comforted Bathsheba his wife, and went in to her and lay with her. So she bore a son, and he called his name Solomon" (12:24, NKJV). Such lovemaking is rich with compassion and love . . . no wonder it brings solace!

Janette told us that when her husband was in despair over losing his job, the most effective comfort and encouragement she gave him was to love him physically. Shelly, married to an intense man, said that when her husband had spent his day at the office slaying dragons with little success, she knew she could comfort him and help him relax by making love to him. Ginny shared this touching account with us:

> My husband was heaped in a chair, deeply discouraged. A friend had betrayed him. "Honey, take off your shirt and lie on the bed. I've got

hot oil and am going to massage the tension out of your muscles."
As I rubbed his shoulders and back, I could feel his tension evaporate. I took off his remaining clothes and massaged the rest of his
body. Then I comforted him with my love. It wasn't a sensuous time
of lovemaking or a glorious time of intimate oneness. It was a time
of giving comfort. When he sighed deeply and fell asleep, I felt such
joy because of the love I had been able to give.

Lovemaking comforts because it releases tension. A backrub is good for
tense bodies, a sexual release even better. God was ingenious in His creation. Through our lovemaking we can create life, experience one-flesh
intimacy and deep knowledge, enjoy deep pleasure, and even comfort each
other in times of stress or sorrow.

LISTEN TO GOD'S VOICE

The world has desecrated God's beautiful gift of sex. What He made pure,
the world putrefied. What He made sacred, the world made sleazy. What the
world did was wrong, but a wife is just as wrong if she allows the world's des-
ecration to keep her from embracing the beauty of God's viewpoint. God
desires that a husband and wife be naked and unashamed, glorying in the
giving and receiving of exquisite pleasure and rejoicing in the intimate oneness that sex brings.

Wherever you are today, be assured that God is a God who redeems. He
longs to show you that His gift can be erotic, fulfilling, free, and beautiful. But
in order for you to enjoy the sexual relationship within your marriage, you have
to throw out the mental tapes which play any message that conflicts with
God's voice. You need to hear His voice alone; you need to listen to the One
Voice. Our gracious God will speak to you. He longs to help you. And if you
ask, He will redeem His beautiful gift in your life and make all things new.

> *God, I choose to close my ears to the voices of the world and listen to*
> *You. I trust You to heal where healing is needed, to teach me where I*
> *lack wisdom, and to direct me as I seek to enjoy intimacy with my*
> *husband. I surrender myself to You and ask You to redeem Your beau-*
> *tiful gift of sex in my life.*

CHANGE MY HEART, O GOD

We don't need to seek the world's viewpoint on sex in order to know it. It shouts at us from billboards, television, radio, newspapers—even the packaging on the products we buy. But to know God's viewpoint of sex, we must seek it.

1. Listed below are three ways you can better understand God's view of sex. Choose at least one you intend to pursue.

    ✒ Read and meditate on the Song of Solomon.

    ✒ Pick either Proverbs 5:15-19 or 1 Corinthians 7:2,5 to meditate on, and write what you feel God is teaching you about sex in this passage.

    ✒ Continue reading in this book and ask God to reveal His viewpoint on sex.

2. Of the six reasons why God gave the gift of sex, which one did you find most encouraging? How can this viewpoint affect your sexual relationship with your husband?

3. What one thing can you do this week to incorporate this viewpoint into your own way of thinking?

two

How Can I Be Godly *and* Sensuous?

*O*ne of the most thought-provoking stories from those we surveyed came from a woman named Heidi. She asked her husband, Brent, what he would like for his birthday present. She expected him to say something ordinary like new golf clubs. Instead, his extraordinary request stunned her: "Honey, the only gift I desire is for you to give yourself permission to be a sensuous woman." Heidi's eyes filled with tears. *Give myself permission? Become a sensuous woman? What does he mean?*

Like Heidi, many Christian women believe that sex is a gift from God, but even so, they can't give themselves permission to revel in the sensuous pleasures of married love. Why? Because in their minds, the words *godly* and *sensuous* do not go together. Their definition of a godly woman does not include words like *sexual* or *sensuous,* and so in their quest to become godly women, they have denied their sensuousness. As a result, they are withholding from both their husbands and themselves one of God's greatest gifts: the ability to *delight* in their physical union with their husbands.

When we asked fifteen pastors' wives for their definitions of a godly wife, we heard many good answers, including:

> "She fears the Lord, is transparent, and possesses a gentle and quiet spirit."

> "She is a woman who loves her husband and children, is full of wisdom and obedient."

> "She is joyful and content; strength and dignity characterize her."

Did you notice what's missing? None of these answers contain anything that could be considered physical. Only spiritual qualities were mentioned.

Most Christian women believe that God created them to be sexual and that He fashioned their body to fit with their husband's body in a wondrous way. But even knowing God's perspective, they can't give themselves permission to be sensuous. Perhaps one reason is because they view the word *sensuous* in a negative way.

Webster defines *sensuous* as "pertaining to the senses; appealing to the senses, alive to the pleasure to be received through the senses." *Sensuous* is a positive term. *Sensual*, on the other hand, is most often used in the negative, referring to an unrestrained sexual appetite, which is always wrong and ungodly (Galatians 5:19). Throughout this book *sensuous* will be used as a positive term—to be "alive to the pleasure to be received through the senses" *with your husband.* This is exactly what God wants for us.

We've asked many women: "Do you give yourselves permission to be a sensuous wife?" Their responses varied. Some women who married later in life have spent so many years "damming up" their sexual passions in an attempt to remain pure that they find it difficult suddenly to open the floodgates and allow sexual feelings to flow. They have ignored their sexuality so long that it has atrophied. Others are unable to forgive themselves for past sexual sin and feel part of their penance must be never to enjoy sex "too much" (see chapter 8). But the most common reason is that the world has so drastically perverted God's gift of sex that many women feel they have to disassociate themselves from anything erotic or sensuous in order to be godly.

It's as if everything related to sex gets tossed into one soup pot and is stirred together. We poke through the soup and pick out what is disagreeable, but even after it's gone, we have a bad taste in our mouth. Rather than delighting in the mouth-watering soup God urges us to eat, we throw out the whole pot and deny our hunger.

ARE YOU LIVING IN "TWO STORIES"?

What happens when we discard what God created for the sake of a few rotten carrots? Sex with our husband becomes routine and passionless. We do not allow ourselves to feel wild abandonment or erotic pleasure because that would be *too* much like the world. We divert the passion we might otherwise enjoy in sexual intimacy with our husbands into other ventures such as work, children, or spiritual growth.

Leslie, while listless in bed, is passionate when it comes to her relationship with God. "The more I grow as a Christian, the less important the physical becomes. I want my emphasis to be on the spiritual," Leslie says. She justifies her thinking with scriptures such as: "Live by the Spirit, and you will not gratify the desires of the sinful nature" (Galatians 5:16, NIV) and "Set your minds on things above, not on earthly things" (Colossians 3:2, NIV).

Unfortunately, Leslie has misinterpreted the scriptures. She has associated *desire* and *earthly* in these verses with sexual pleasures, when in reality they refer to selfish pursuits. Leslie's spiritual idealism conflicted with the realities of physical living. She was a physical being in a physical world; how could she stay spiritual? Her solution was to separate the two realms. Physical things, such as sex, went into one compartment; spiritual things went into another. In her passion to become a godly woman, Leslie became a divided woman.

Many women fall into this trap. As one woman put it: "It's as if I live in a two-story house. The top floor is my spirituality and the bottom floor my sexuality. In between the two floors is a brick barrier separating my spiritual self from my sexual self. Because I want to be godly, I can't allow myself to be too earthly—and sex is definitely earthly. I allow myself to experience pleasure—but only so much. If I got really carried away, it would be 'too fleshly.'"

Dear friend, this ought not to be. When God created us female, He integrated our sexuality with our spirituality. He meant for the spiritual and sexual to melt together. Why else would God take the ultimate sexual act, sexual intercourse between a husband and wife, and liken it to the ultimate spiritual experience, the union of Christ and the church (Ephesians 5:31-32)? Just as a husband and wife experience deep joy as they lose themselves and merge into oneness at the moment of sexual climax, we experience ultimate joy as we become one with Jesus Christ in a union that leads to incomprehensible joy. Sexual intercourse mirrors our relationship to God and causes us to worship Him for giving us this good gift.[1]

Spiritual intimacy and delight are not in opposition to sexual intimacy and delight. Spiritual intimacy is actually found in the midst of the relational, fleshly delight of sexual union. Drs. Dan Allender and Tremper Longman, in their excellent book *Intimate Allies*, say that "a taste of the character of God is found in sexual foreplay, heightened arousal, orgasm, and quiescence. God is a God of passion. He adores joy, and he delights in our delight in glory."[2]

GOD DECLARES: "BE WHOLE"

God beckons us and says, "Be clothed with my perspective." "For everything created by God is good, and nothing is to be rejected, if it is received with gratitude; for it is sanctified by means of the word of God and prayer" (1 Timothy 4:4-5). Did you hear what God declares? EVERYTHING is GOOD and NOTHING is to be rejected if we receive it with thanksgiving. The word *everything* includes sexuality! "For everything [including your sexuality] comes from God alone. Everything [including your sexuality] lives by his power, and everything [including your sexuality] is for his glory. To him be glory evermore" (Romans 11:36, TLB).

Everything encompasses EVERYTHING. William Newell in his commentary on Romans says that *everything* includes our minds, our spirits, and our bodies.[3] All of life—what we look like, our gifts, talents, faith, possessions, husband, children, jobs, *and* our sexuality—all come from God alone and all is for His glory. When we live "in a two-story house" and separate our spirituality from our sexuality, we divide what God made whole. We intimate that God's gift of sex is not good enough—not worthy to be placed alongside the spiritual.

Many women have thanked God that He knit them together in their mother's wombs, that He made them fearfully and wonderfully (Psalm 139:13-14). They can continue to say with David, "Wonderful are Thy works, and my soul knows it very well" (Psalm 139:14). But they fail to acknowledge that their sexuality is part of their physical makeup. Have you ever thanked God that when He knit your physical makeup together, part of His beautiful embroidery was your sexuality?

Our sexuality and spirituality are not separate and divided, as are the top and bottom floors in a two-story house. Rather, they form a circle, whole and unbroken. Vonette Bright beautifully describes the circle of our spirituality and sexuality: "It is as important to be filled with the Spirit in bed with your husband, ministering to him, as it is for you to be filled with the Spirit when you are teaching the Bible or ministering."[4]

Perhaps the most powerful illustration of the union of the sexual and the spiritual is found in the Song of Solomon. In these verses God paints an astounding picture. Solomon and Shulamith[5] are engaged in steamy, erotic, sensuous lovemaking. Suddenly, a third Person appears in the room: God. Tenderly, the Almighty Creator gazes upon the naked lovers engaged in physical pleasures and extends His hand in spiritual blessing: "Eat, friends; drink and imbibe deeply, O lovers" (Song of Solomon 5:1).

Imagine! God is there. He sees the passion. He hears the sighs of delight. He watches the lovers as they caress one another in the most intimate places. He is witness to the fleshly, earthy sights, sounds, and smells. He sees it all and then urges the lovers to feast, to drink abundantly of the exquisite pleasures He created for them to enjoy.

God desires for us to rejoice in our sensuousness, to give in to it. He wants us to hold nothing back, to open the floodgates of physical passion and immerse ourselves in it. "Drink and imbibe deeply," He urges.

Perhaps you are thinking, *I can give myself permission to go deeper in my sexuality because I see now that this is part of who God created me to be. But I'm not sure how this translates practically. What do I do? How should I act? What does a godly, sensuous woman look like?*

Graciously, God provides an answer in His Word.

WHO AM I AS A SENSUOUS, SEXUAL WOMAN?

In Scripture God holds up examples for us to follow as we seek to display His character and be conformed to His image. If, for example, we desire to grow in the attribute of loyalty, we might want to look at Ruth. If we seek to forgive others, Joseph shows us the way. If, however, we desire to grow in our sensuousness as wives, we can study and emulate Solomon's bride, Shulamith.

Turn with us to the Song of Solomon, a beautiful book that describes the courtship, wedding, and early years of King Solomon's marriage to Shulamith. It is written in a poetic style called lyric idyll and contains a series of fifteen reflections by Shulamith. It unfolds like a movie with several flashbacks, the story being temporarily suspended while the audience views a scene from the past. This explains the lack of chronological sequence in the Song.[6] It also explains why many couples who read this book find it confusing! But the nuggets of gold hidden in this book are worth digging for. Let's look at the portrait of Shulamith as a godly and sensuous woman.

She is responsive. Shulamith whispers longingly in Solomon's ear: "Make my garden breathe out fragrance, let its spices be wafted abroad. May my beloved come into his garden and eat its choice fruits!" (4:16).

She is adventurous. At times Shulamith receives sexual pleasure from her husband. Other times she is the initiator, aggressively stimulating her lover through intoxicating fragrances, seductive sights, and the promise of sexual ecstasy. This clever wife titillates her husband by suggesting they take a vacation together in the country and make love outdoors. There among the vineyards, she will offer him old sexual delicacies and new sexual delights (7:11-13).

She is uninhibited. Shulamith tells her husband where to touch her so she will become sexually aroused (2:6, 4:16). She tantalizes him with sexual treats that make his mouth water, enticing him with her body. Her sensuousness reaches an apex when she performs an erotic nude dance, provocatively sway-ing her hips before him as an invitation to lovemaking (7:1-3).

She is expressive. Shulamith is verbally expressive: "My beloved is mine and I am his" (2:16). She expresses praise for her husband's masculinity: "How handsome you are, my beloved" (1:16). "Like an apple tree among the trees of the forest, so is my beloved among the young men" (2:3).

She is sensuous. A sensuous woman is tuned in to her body and the stimulation she receives through her five senses. She delights in her senses. In Song of Solomon 5:10-16, Shulamith gives in to her sexuality and thinks about her husband in very sensuous terms. Solomon is not present, and Shulamith meditates on her husband's body, describing him with erotic imagery. In her mind she undresses her husband, beginning at the top of his head and working her way downward. She dwells on his sensu-ous lips, his muscular shoulders, and strong legs and ends her daydreaming by saying: "His mouth is full of sweetness. And he is wholly desirable" (5:16). Shulamith's thoughts prepared her to act out her sensuousness with her husband.

No doubt about it, Shulamith was a sensuous, sexual woman—and God describes her sensuousness in explicit and erotic terms. God wants us to understand the beauty and freedom of our sexuality. Through the young bride Shulamith, God unveils the portrait of a godly, sensuous wife and, because His blessing is upon her, we can follow her example with confidence.

If you are thinking, *I could never be like that,* don't be discouraged. God does not expect us to become sensuous saints overnight. He asks instead that we go forward in becoming the lovers He created us to be. Christian women should be the greatest lovers on earth because, as believers, we not only possess physical passion, we have the ability to infuse holiness into our sensuousness.

PRAY FOR A NEW BEGINNING

If you are ready to begin the metamorphosis and blossom into all God created you to be, the place to start enacting change is not in the bedroom but on your knees. Changed actions are the result of changed attitudes. Changed attitudes begin with prayer. Won't you pray now and ask God to work in your heart and mind?

GROWING IN GODLY SENSUOUSNESS

Beth: "Loving my husband can become an act of worship to God.

"As my husband and I lie together, satiated in the afterglow of sexual ecstasy, the most natural thing in the world is for me to offer thanksgiving to my God for the beauty, the glory of our sexual joy. I don't even think about what I am doing; my heart just turns to the Lord and offers praise. Truly His gift of sex is a wondrous thing."

Courtney: "I finally gave myself permission to be sensuous.

"I had been married for four months. One day I experienced an overwhelming love for God, and it occurred to me that sexual pleasure was created for ME. I knew God had planned sex, that it was His gift, but I hadn't appropriated His gift personally. I gave myself permission to be sensuous. It was a night my husband won't soon forget . . . nor will I. I became an actress in the play, not just someone who 'showed up.' If I'm part of the play, I set up the props and am involved in setting the stage, and what a difference it makes!"

Pray: "God, give me a new mind." Your mind must be reprogrammed with new information. All the voices that shout, "Don't be sensuous," must be replaced with God's voice. He not only gives you permission to be sensuous, He encourages it! Memorize Song of Solomon 5:1: "Eat, friends; drink and imbibe deeply, O lovers." Ask God to make His perspective, your perspective. Thank Him that, even now, He is renewing your mind (Romans 12:2).

Pray: "God, give me an undivided heart." Jesus warns in Luke 11:17 (NIV), "A house divided against itself will fall." God desires that we reclaim the pleasure of our bodies as much as we are to reclaim the purity of our souls.[7] He longs for us to be whole women, not divided women who separate our spirituality and sexuality. Listen to God's promise through the prophet Ezekiel: "I will give them an undivided heart and put a new spirit in them; I will remove from them their heart of stone and give them a heart of flesh" (11:19, NIV). If we separate our spiritual self from our sexual self, it's as if we have a heart of stone, a heart with a brick barrier between the "two stories" of our being. But God says He will remove the stone. He promises to put His spirit in our flesh and give us an undivided heart. All we have to do is ask.

Pray: "God, help me be the sensuous lover you created me to be." God intends for us to experience sexual pleasure, to invigorate our senses and draw our hearts to shout with gratitude and praise to God.[8] To accept and delight in the sensuous is to be enraptured by the gifts of God.

God gives us permission to be sensuous. Will you give yourself permission?

If you still feel reluctant, read through the first two chapters again. Allow the truths of God's Word to permeate your heart and mind. Once God's blessing on sensuous love sinks into your thinking, put these revelations into action. Invite your husband to make love with you. As you caress his face, look into his eyes and *feel* the warmth of his body next to yours and praise God for giving you the ability to express physical and spiritual love through intimate touching. Then, as you come together as one, imagine God standing by your bed, His glorious Presence filling the room. See His loving smile. Feel the touch of His hand of blessing. Hear His voice proclaim: "Imbibe deeply, O lovers" (Song of Solomon 5:1).

God, thank you for placing your hand of blessing on our intimate lovemaking. Thank you that you have told us to feast on our sexual joy, to revel in the exquisite feelings that you created. I desire to begin to deeply taste of the sexual joy you have for me. I yield to your Spirit! Teach me to become the sensuous woman you created me to be.

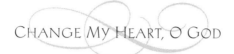

CHANGE MY HEART, O GOD

1. Are you living in a two-story house with a brick wall separating your sexuality from your spirituality? What are the bricks in your barrier?

2. How can the bricks that separate your sexuality from your spirituality be removed?

3. Memorize Romans 11:36. Thank God that your sexuality is included in "all things."

4. What step will you take this week in response to what God has shown you in this chapter? (Read again the portrait of Shulamith, a sensuous woman.)

three

How Do I Shift into Sexual Gear?

*I*n C. S. Lewis's popular Chronicles of Narnia, four children climb into an old wardrobe and discover a hidden door that allows them to enter a new world brimming with unimaginable adventures and never-before-seen possibilities.

For many, reading this book has placed you before a similar kind of door. Behind it is a new world filled with godly—yet unimaginable—sexual pleasures and adventures.

In chapter 1, we cracked open the door and peeked into this new world as we considered God's intended purpose for physical intimacy. In chapter 2, we nudged the door open further as we discovered God's perspective as revealed in the godly and sensuous Shulamith. In this chapter, we will fling wide the door and bravely venture out into this glorious new world. Lift your eyes. Gaze into the distance. Unexpected pleasures await you. A path will take you there. That path is your mind.

Many women are surprised when we tell them that the mind is the most important sexual organ. It's true. The mind is the command center for all sexual feelings. It's the congress that governs your sexual state. It is the storehouse for every sexual thought you've ever had. According to Dr. Douglas Rosenau, theologian and Christian sex therapist, "Sex is 80 percent imagination and mind and 20 percent friction."[1]

This small organ weighs just over three pounds, but it has 12 billion cells and 120 trillion connections. If the mind were a computer, it would be the size of the Empire State Building![2] Ten thousand thoughts go through the human mind in one day. These thoughts determine who we are, what we do, and who we will become. Proverbs 23:7 says, "As a woman thinks within herself, so shall she be" (our paraphrase). Ralph Waldo Emerson said it like this: "Beware of what you set your mind on for that you will surely become." We become what we think—so obviously what we think is important!

How do you think of yourself as a lover? Some women see themselves as "godly and sensuous;" others say they feel like a threadbare dishrag, limp and frayed with no enthusiasm for lovemaking. We would encourage you to be eager to learn more about how to enhance your sexual relationship with your husband. Even after years of marriage, you can continue to be innovative and creative—it's all in how you think. The more sexual your thoughts about your husband, the more pleasurable your lovemaking.

But in talking with women about this subject, we've learned that many don't consciously try to use their minds to enhance their sexual relationship. As we've noted, some, as Christians, don't feel comfortable; others have simply never considered it. Mark this down: You are what you think, and how you think about sex greatly affects your relationship with your husband. If you view sex as neutral or negative, you can make it positive by changing the way you think. Let's put it another way:

> Major Premise: We can control our thoughts.
>
> Minor Premise: Our feelings come from our thoughts.
>
> Conclusion: We can control our feelings by learning to change one thing, the way we think.[3]

MINDING YOUR MIND

Most of us are better about controlling our bodies than we are about controlling our minds. We allow the ten thousand thoughts of the day to trample unrestrained through our heads. Like disobedient children, they race this way and that, generating chaos and a myriad of emotions. This ought not to be, God says. He gave us our minds with the expectation that we were to rule them. He wants us to make our minds mind. God wants us, like a mother wagging her finger at a disobedient child, to tell our thoughts where they can and cannot go. God desires us to nourish certain thoughts and rebuke others saying, "NO! I will NOT go in this direction."

Second Corinthians 10:5 says, "We are destroying speculations and every lofty thing raised up against the knowledge of God, and we are taking every thought captive to the obedience of Christ." We paraphrase this verse as "Don't allow wrong thinking to sit on the throne of your mind. Hurl it down from its lofty position. Throw it into the trash and burn it. As for the good thoughts, lasso them; pull them in. Get your arms around them and make them your own." According to this verse, we must continually choose which thoughts will reign in our minds: right thoughts or wrong thoughts, God's thoughts or the world's thoughts, holy thoughts or sinful thoughts.

"Set your mind on the things above, not on the things that are on earth" (Colossians 3:2). In this passage, the Greek word for *mind* means "a way of thinking" or "mind-set."[4] A mind-set is a collection of individual thoughts that over a period of time influence the way we perceive life. Stop for a moment and ask yourself an important question: How have my individual thoughts over the past twenty years contributed to the sexual mind-set I have today?

Our past experiences, what we were told or not told about sex, what voices we listen to, what we have chosen to embrace and reject, all influence our mind-set. Consider the very different mind-set of three wives.

"I really don't care much for sex. It just seems too worldly and fleshly. I don't want to be like those lustful, panting, immoral women in the movies. I know my husband needs sex, so I'll oblige him. But I'd be happier if sex wasn't a focus in our marriage."

"I am not excited about sex, I guess you could say I feel 'blah' about it. It's always the same and I guess it will be for the rest of our married life."

"I am ready to embrace my sensuousness in a new way! Recently I've realized the freedom and intense pleasure that God intended for a husband and wife in their sexual relationship, and I'm ready for it!"

If you identify with the first or second woman, you need a different mind-set—you need to transform your mind. Romans 12:2 (NIV) says, "Do not conform any longer to the pattern of this world, but be transformed by the renewing of your mind." The word for transformed is the Greek word *metamorphousthe,* from which we get our English word *metamorphosis.* Metamorphosis involves total change, from the inside out.

How Do Your Flowers Grow?

To better understand how you can transform your mind, picture your mind as a flower bed. When you were born, the soil of your mind was bare. As you grew, your life experiences scattered seeds across the flower bed. Some seeds grew into graceful lilies, uplifting ideas which, when nurtured, blossomed into fragrant thoughts. Other seeds produced weeds—thorny, water-sapping lies that robbed the flowers of nourishment. If these lies were not uprooted, they spread and took over entire sections of your mind.

Survey the flower bed in your mind as it relates to sex. Do lovely roses grow there? Or is it a place of disorder, overrun with creeping vines and thorny brambles?

We transform our mind the same way we transform a garden. First, uproot any and all weeds of wrong thinking that choke out the beauty of your garden. Second, plant the flowers of God's perspective that will enhance the grandeur of your flower bed and cause it to flourish. For some, transformation could happen quickly. For others, it may be a long process. Let's take a look at what is involved according to Romans 12:2.

1. Uproot the weeds: "Do not be conformed to this world." In this verse we are told to weed out the world's mind-set which includes lies, immoral acts, and wrong attitudes. Do any of these weeds grow in the garden of your mind?

> Coarse jesting or crude sexual remarks (Ephesians 4:29 says yank these suckers out!)

> Impure thoughts about men (Matthew 5:28 suggests douse with weed-killer.)

Unholy sexual images from past experiences (Isaiah 43:18-19, uproot immediately.)

Selfish attitudes about sex (Philippians 2:3, toss in the trash.)

Negative thoughts about your sexual relationship with your husband (Philippians 4:8, vigorously chop with garden hoe.)

Diligently search your mind for these weeds. Once you've uprooted them, your mind will be ready for flowers to grow in the now vacant places.

2. Plant flower seeds: "Be transformed by the renewing of your mind." Now that the weeds are gone, it's time to plant the seeds of Scripture so that beautiful flowers can bloom. Here are a few seeds to plant, each of which will add color and beauty to your sexual mind-set.

As a loving hind and a graceful doe, let [my] breasts satisfy you at all times; be exhilarated always with [my] love. (Proverbs 5:19)

His mouth is full of sweetness. And he is wholly desirable. This is my beloved and this is my friend. (Song of Solomon 5:16)

I am my beloved's, and his desire is for me. (Song of Solomon 7:10)

Ask God to open your eyes to other seeds that will transform your mind.

Nourish to Flourish

Burying the seeds in the soil is only the first step to growing a beautiful garden. If flowers are to flourish, you must water and fertilize what has been planted. Likewise, after planting the seeds of Scripture in your mind, nourish what you have planted through the disciplines of memorization and meditation.

Memorizing Scripture increases the Holy Spirit's vocabulary in your life.[5] Memorizing is never easy, but it is necessary for true transformation to take place. Write the verses you desire to plant in your mind on note cards and go over them often. Tape them to your bathroom mirror or slip them under your pillow and review them before you go to sleep.

Meditation sends the roots of Scripture down deep as you personalize what you've memorized and pray it back to God. For example, you can meditate on Proverbs 5:19 by praying:

> *God, thank You that You say I am to be like a graceful and beauti-*
> *ful deer to my husband, that my breasts are to satisfy him at all times.*
> *God, show me how to be a creative and sensuous lover to him, how*
> *to use my breasts, my body to give him pleasure. I want him to be*
> *intoxicated and exhilarated with my skill as a lover.*

When we memorize and meditate on God's Word, new thought patterns blossom in our minds. As the new mind-set filters down to the recesses of the heart, we begin to act differently. We are more willing to step out of our comfort zone and try new things.

I (Linda) remember making a choice to be more expressive in my love-making in the early years of our marriage. I was glad I had memorized and meditated on the passages in Song of Solomon. I was ready to take some new actions, but when my husband, Jody, asked me to describe in detail everything I was going to do to pleasure him sexually, I said (gulp), "In detail?" How could I do this? What words would I use? At the time, it took every bit of nerve I had to grant this desire, but I did it.

The first time we try something new, it's always difficult. With time, however, it gets easier. Like stepping into a cold lake, at first our body feels shock. But with each step, we get used to the water until, pretty soon, we enjoy a refreshing swim.

Take a step. Be expressive as a lover. Take a step. Try a new position. Take a step. Make love in a new location. Take a step. Allow your mind to dwell on your husband's body. This is what Shulamith did.

LET YOUR MIND GO

Shulamith, a biblical example of a godly and sensuous wife, used her mind to shift into sexual gear. She had placed a storehouse of treasured erotic memories in her mind and here we see her pulling one out and reliving it. She is thinking about her lover, Solomon, in very sensuous ways. Listen to her beautiful words:

My beloved is dazzling and ruddy, outstanding among ten thousand. His head is like gold, pure gold; his locks are like clusters of dates, and black as a raven. His eyes are like doves, beside streams of water, bathed in milk, and reposed in their setting. His cheeks are like a bed of balsam, banks of sweet-scented herbs; his lips are lilies, dripping with liquid myrrh. His hands are rods of gold set with beryl; his abdomen is carved ivory inlaid with sapphires. His legs are pillars of alabaster set on pedestals of pure gold; his appearance is like Lebanon, choice as the cedars. His mouth is full of sweetness. And he is wholly desirable. This is my beloved and this is my friend, O daughters of Jerusalem. (Song of Solomon 5:10-16)

Beginning with the head and face of her beloved, Shulamith lets her mind slowly undress him as she moves down his body. The authors of *Intimate Allies,* one of whom is an Old Testament scholar, make this statement about the nature of her thinking:

After commenting on his strong arms, she then describes a part of his body as polished ivory. Most English translations hesitate in this verse. The Hebrew is quite erotic, and most translators cannot bring themselves to bring out the obvious meaning. The smooth and expensively ornamented tusk of ivory is a loving description of her husband's erect penis.[6]

Are you surprised that God included in His Holy Word a picture of a wife imagining her husband's naked body? (Note the important word *husband.* It is your husband's body you are to dwell on, not something you read in a romantic novel or view on a movie screen.)

God not only gives us permission to dwell on our husband's body, He encourages it. He seems to say, "Your husband's body is a work of art that I created. Dwell on every inch of him and marvel at how he is fashioned, from the tip of his head to his toes." Let your mind go when it comes to fantasizing about your husband. Such thinking will prepare your heart and body for lovemaking.

Dr. Rosenau, author of *A Celebration of Sex,* says, "Our mind and the ability to think and imagine are a crucial part of being created human. This ability to enjoy mental imagery can be used to expand and enjoy all aspects of your life, including lovemaking."[7] Dear friend, fill the storehouse of your mind with treasured memories of your husband.

Pam said she and her husband spent one evening sharing their favorite lovemaking memories. Carol had always thought making love in the rain would be glorious. So instead of dreaming about it, she took her husband out in their backyard one night in a thunderstorm and created her own memory.

We pray your mind has been stretched because a stretched mind will never snap back into its original shape. We urge you to continue to uproot the weeds of wrong thinking and plant the seeds of Scripture. "Whatever is true, whatever is noble, whatever is right, whatever is pure, whatever is lovely, whatever is admirable—if anything is excellent or praiseworthy— think about such things" (Philippians 4:8, NIV).

It is right, pure, and holy to daydream about your husband's body.

It is right, pure, and holy to train your mind to help you shift into sexual gear.

It is right, pure, and holy to store up a treasure chest of sexual memories of your beloved.

The right sexual thoughts become actions which eventually become habits and new attitudes.[8]

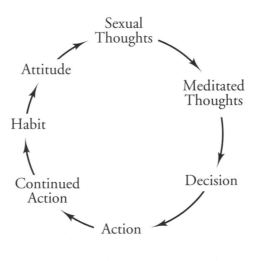

Marcus Aurelius said, "Our life is what our thoughts make it." We would add, "Our sexual life is what our thoughts make it." Your mind is your greatest sexual organ. Use it to become the godly and sensuous lover God desires you to be!

CHANGE MY HEART, O GOD

1. Make a list of wrong sexual thoughts God wants you to "uproot" from your mind. Confess them one by one to God. Then tear up the list and throw the pieces of paper into the trash.

2. Make a list of right sexual thoughts from Scripture that God wants to implant in your mind. (Refer to pages 26-7.) Say each one aloud to God. Tell Him you want a new mind-set. Keep this list in a private place, and review it often.

3. Pick two verses to memorize from the Song of Solomon. After you have planted them in your memory, meditate on them and pray them back to God. Then ask God if you need to step out and "make a choice" based on these verses.

4. Review how Shulamith used imagery to shift her mind into sexual gear. (See pages 28-30.) Ask God to show you how you can use your mind in a similar way.

How Can I Relate When He's a Microwave and I'm a Crockpot?

*W*hen both of us were in high school, boys played sports and girls stood on the sidelines and cheered. As our teams marched down the football field toward the goal line, we used to chant: "Lean to the left. Lean to the right. Stand up. Sit down. Fight! Fight! Fight!"

This cheer aptly summarizes how society has viewed the differences between men and women over the last century. In the early 1900s, women didn't discuss politics. Men didn't help in the kitchen. Men loved sex. Women tolerated sex. Men and women were viewed as DIFFERENT . . . *lean to the left.*

In the 1970s, the feminist movement marched on the scene. Women wanted equal roles, equal pay, equal orgasm. Men and women struggled to be viewed as the SAME . . . *lean to the right.*

Today as we approach the twenty-first century, it's *lean to the left* again as men and women are viewed as so different that, according to best-selling author Dr. John Gray, men come from Mars and women come from Venus. Back and forth society swings in the unending debate. Are we different? Are we the same?

Actually both statements are true. Men and women are similar in their need for love, admiration, and respect. We are alike in our desire to find meaning and purpose in life and our need for physical and emotional love. But we are also very different, especially when it comes to sex.

The purpose of this chapter is to discuss the sexual differences between men and women and to see how these differences can help build a stronger sexual relationship. Such a discussion should start at the beginning—the very beginning when God created the first man and the first woman. Let's visit the creation account and see what it can tell us about the differences between the sexes.

GOD CREATED US TO BE DIFFERENT

You've probably read the following verses from Genesis a gazillion times, so ask God to help you see them with fresh eyes. Read slowly. Make a mental notation of the created differences between man and woman. Then compare your list to ours.

> The LORD God formed the man from the dust of the ground and breathed into his nostrils the breath of life, and the man became a living being. . . . The LORD God took the man and put him in the Garden of Eden to work it and take care of it. (2:7,15, NIV)

> The LORD God said, "It is not good for the man to be alone. I will make a helper suitable for him." (2:18, NIV)

> Now the LORD God had formed out of the ground all the beasts of the field and all the birds of the air. He brought them to the man to see what he would name them. . . . But for Adam no suitable helper was found. (2:19-20, NIV)

> So the LORD God caused the man to fall into a deep sleep; and while he was sleeping, he took one of the man's ribs and closed up the place with flesh. Then the LORD God made a woman from the rib he had taken out of the man, and he brought her to the man. The man said, "This is now bone of my bones and flesh of my flesh; she shall be called 'woman,' for she was taken out of man." (2:21-23, NIV)

> Adam named his wife Eve, because she would become the mother of all the living. (3:20, NIV)

Based on these verses, here's our list of male/female differences:

➤ Man was formed from dust; woman was formed from flesh.

- ❧ Man was placed in the garden alone; woman was brought to the man so they could be together.
- ❧ Man was created with a need; woman was created to fill a need.
- ❧ Man's job was to work; woman's job was to help man with his work.
- ❧ Man's job was cognitive/task oriented (name the animals); woman's job was emotive/relational (meet the need of the man).
- ❧ Man gave woman her name; woman received her name from man.
- ❧ Man's body was created to give a seed; woman's body was created to give life.

God created man and woman with different physical features, gave them different abilities, and assigned them different roles. Then He created an avenue in which all their differences could melt away. In the intimacy of sexual love, differences dissolved, and the two separate and distinctly different individuals became one flesh (2:24).

What God designed was holy and right. The differences He fashioned are an asset, not a liability. Only together—with all their differences—can man and woman accomplish God's purposes and picture God and His people.

God's original intent was that man and woman would dwell together, work together, complete one another, and enjoy the ecstasy of marital love. But sin entered the picture and slashed the couple's oneness. Immediately "their eyes were opened." Instead of being naked and unashamed, Adam and Eve hid their bodies. Instead of being grateful for each other, they blamed one another. Their differences no longer united them, but divided them. Even the beauty of sex did not always bring about the original oneness they had known in the beginning.

Can we return to the beauty of love that God originally intended? Yes. Proverbs 24:3-4 says, "By wisdom a house is built, and by understanding it is established; and by knowledge the rooms are filled with all precious and pleasant riches." This principle can be applied to our sexual relationship: We must seek wisdom, understanding, and knowledge about the ways in which our spouse is different from us, and then use this information to dissolve differences and regain oneness.

SIX DIFFERENCES THAT AFFECT INTIMACY

From the moment of conception, chromosomes encode femininity or masculinity into every fiber of our being. As a result, men and women differ in every cell of their bodies. A man's muscular and skeletal structure tends to be larger and stronger than a woman's. In brute strength, men are 50 percent above women.[1] A woman's heart generally beats faster than a man's (eighty versus seventy-two), and her blood pressure is lower (on average, about ten points). This is how God made us.

Because of the differences in their physical makeup, men and women respond differently to sex. We want to highlight six questions women often ask that express some frustration or lack of understanding about their man. Each of these questions stem from the physiological differences between men and women, differences that impact the sexual relationship. But first, we'd like to wave a red flag of disclaimer. Some of the information that follows may fit you well; some may not. We are well aware that while there are differences *between* the sexes, there are also differences *among* the sexes. No two women are alike. No two men are alike. As you read, ask God to give you wisdom, to increase your understanding and knowledge so that you may uncover the precious riches hidden in these words that are meant for you and your husband.

WHY CAN HE ONLY FOCUS ON ONE THING AT A TIME?

In the womb, a male baby is subjected to a "testosterone bath" sometime between the sixteenth and twenty-sixth weeks of development.[2] In addition to accentuating masculine traits in the child, this "bath" severs some of the connecting nerve endings between the left and right hemispheres of the brain. As a result, men find it more difficult to switch between left- and right-brain functions. Since women are not subjected to this bath, their connecting fibers remain intact, allowing them to switch quickly between the two hemispheres. As a result, a woman tends to think about and do three things at once while a man tends to be single-focused. Simply put, during sex, a husband is focused on the act itself while a wife can enjoy the closeness but at the same time mentally redecorate the bedroom.

The upside of having all our connecting fibers intact is that we can juggle many situations at once. The downside is that we are easily distracted. One husband said, "I hate it when I'm trying to make love to my wife and her mind is a million miles away. She's thinking about a problem with one of the kids or planning tomorrow's dinner menu. I want her to focus on us."

Difference Dissolver: Sex is a time to be single-focused. If you are having trouble getting your mind into sexual gear, read chapter 3. You—and your husband—will be glad you did!

WHY DOES HE SEEM TO HAVE SEX ON THE BRAIN?

Hormone levels greatly influence sexual desire. A man is like a river. His testosterone levels flow constant and steady. A woman is like an ocean. Her hormones ebb and flow, depending on where she is in her menstrual cycle. In the early part of her cycle when estrogen levels are high, desire for sex can wash over her with the force of a typhoon. Several days later, after ovulation, she may want nothing to do with sex—ever again.

A man may have sex on the brain, but the part of his body he wants touched is approximately forty inches south. A man's sexual glands are concentrated in one location, his genitals. But that one location contains so many stimulation points that even a mild touch drives him wild. A man has seventeen sexual glands. Like millions of Energizer Bunnies, these glands work day and night, producing semen, which is stored in an inner sac in the testes. When the sac fills up, his testes tell his brain, "Do something quick before I explode!" A man's need for sex is not all in his mind; his sexual command center demands release from the accumulated buildup.

Contrast this to a woman's body. Every inch of the female anatomy can trigger sexual longing. A caress in the small of her back, a lingering hand on her thigh, a slow stroke on her arm can all send tingles to the tips of her toes. And we haven't even mentioned the hot spots! These differences could be summarized like this: A woman responds to accumulated touches in many parts of her body until she reaches the desire to be "filled up" while a man quickly responds to direct touch of his genitals and feels a need to "empty out."

Difference Dissolver: A wise woman charts her cycle and rides the wave of desire by initiating sex with her husband when her estrogen level is high.

WHY DOES HE CONSIDER A GRUNT MEANINGFUL COMMUNICATION?

Another discernible difference between the sexes is that women generally possess a stronger need for verbal expression than do men. Researchers at Queen's University in Belfast, Northern Ireland, discovered that girl babies move their mouths more than boy babies even before birth. Ultrasounds performed on pregnant women showed that twenty weeks into gestation, girls made about 30 percent more mouth movements per hour than boys.[3] Scripture reinforces this notion. In the Song of Solomon, Shulamith's verbal comments outnumber Solomon's two to one. (This may explain why, during sex, you say, "Oh, honey, that feels so good," and he simply grunts!)

Since women are the verbal queens, we ought to use our skill to build up our spouse. According to one magazine article, "What most men need is reassurance of manhood in addition to sexual gratification."[4] Lauren used her verbal skills to reassure her husband's manhood in a couples' Bible study. Each couple was asked to share one attribute they appreciated most about their spouse. While others responded with comments such as, "her outgoing personality" or "his ability to provide for our family," Lauren said, "What I appreciate most about my husband is that he is a terrific lover." For months after that meeting, the men in the group badgered Lauren's husband. "How did you get her to say that? Tell us your secret."

Difference Dissolver: Next time you and your husband are together, tell him something positive about his prowess as a lover. (If he responds with a grunt, grunt back. You might be surprised to discover how much communication takes place!)

WHY DOES THE SIGHT OF A SHAPELY WOMAN TURN HIS HEAD?

Don't be surprised if your husband looks twice at a sexy redhead in skintight shorts. A man's "optic nerve is directly connected to his penis," according to Dr. Bernie Zilbergeld, author of *The New Male Sexuality.*[5] After we told one woman this, she went home and searched her husband for a hidden wire connecting these two locations. "I couldn't find it," she said, "but I *know* it's there!"

For most men, the connection between an erotic image and sexual arousal is powerful and instantaneous.[6] The bride of Solomon understood this. Remember how she aroused her lover's sexual senses by performing a nude dance before him (Song of Solomon 6:13; 7:1)?

Your husband loves to see your naked body. He enjoys seeing the two of you coming together. This is a gigantic turnon for him. But the biggest "turn on" is to see a look of desire in your eyes.

Difference Dissolver: Are you willing to seductively display your body before your husband? If so, do it! If this is beyond your comfort zone, stimulate his optic nerve by making love in a room filled with mirrors or glowing candles.

WHY IS ORGASM SO EASY FOR HIM?

"My husband turns on quicker than a microwave; I'm more like a slow-cooking Crockpot," Janet said. The difference in the amount of time it takes for a man to achieve orgasm versus a woman is a real one. A man usually needs about two or three minutes of stimulation to have an orgasm, but a woman generally needs ten times that amount of time. Dr. John Gray, author of *Mars and Venus in the Bedroom,* says, "For a woman to experience the big 'O', a man needs to place the 'O' after his two or three minutes, making it twenty to thirty minutes."[7]

Orgasm is different for men than for women. A man's orgasmic feeling is centered primarily in his genitals. For a woman, orgasmic feelings begin in her genitals but send waves throughout the whole body and back to the genitals. When a man reaches "the point of no return," he *must* ejaculate. The house could be on fire, but his "fire" must be put out first! In contrast, a woman's orgasmic response can be broken even after it has begun. Countless wives know the frustration of being on the brink of orgasm when the baby cries or the phone rings, and the edge of ecstasy is lost.

Here are some other ways men and women differ when it comes to orgasms:

- For most men, orgasm is instinctive. For most women it is learned. (We know wives who have never experienced this pleasure. If you are one, chapter 16 is just for you!)
- Men climax easily during intercourse. Most women can't achieve orgasm without direct stimulation of the clitoris.
- A man's climax generally lasts from ten to thirteen seconds. A woman's lasts from six to sixty seconds.[8]
- After orgasm, a man must have a recuperative period. A woman is capable of repeated orgasms with them coming minutes apart or in rapid succession.
- During sex, a man's body releases oxytocin, a hormone thought to cause drowsiness, which makes him want to sleep.[9] While a woman is relaxed after sex, she often wants to stay awake and talk or cuddle.
- "Men have their peak orgasms between ages eighteen to twenty; women soar sexually in their thirties and forties."[10]

Difference Dissolver. Use your verbal skills. Like Shulamith, describe to your husband what feels good to you and where it feels best. Be specific. Be affirmative when he hits the right spots. Share with one another what the buildup of sexual desire feels like and how it feels when the waves of pleasure envelop you.

WHY CAN'T HE JUST CUDDLE?

Cuddling, for a woman, fills an emotional need. When her husband cuddles with his wife, he is saying, "I love you. You are important to me. I love being near you." Sex, for a man, fills this same emotional need. When a wife makes love to her husband, she is saying, "I love you. You are important to me. I love being near you." We women insist that our husbands share their emotions with us. Must we also insist that this sharing be verbal rather than physical?

As women, we sometimes pooh-pooh physical needs because we are masters at dismissing our own physical needs. But we wouldn't dream of dismissing an emotional need. Emotional needs are so—valid! A man has a physical need for sex, but for him, sex also meets a deep emotional need. When you make love to your husband, you touch his soul and create an outlet of expression for his emotions. In essence, touching him enables him to get in touch with himself. Listen to Dr. John Gray's insight:

> Many times after having great sex with my wife, I realize that I had forgotten how beautiful the trees are in our neighborhood. I go outside and breathe in the fresh air and feel alive again. It is not that I didn't feel alive in my work, but by connecting with my wife through great sex, I can reawaken and bring to life my more sensual feelings that are easily forgotten in the focused pursuit of achieving my goals at work. In a sense, great sex helps me to stop and smell the flowers.[11]

Difference Dissolver: Grab your husband's hand and lead him into the bedroom. Tell him you are long overdue for a time of deep, emotional communication. Then proceed to remove your clothes.

VIVA LA DIFFERENCE!

We've discussed seven created differences and six physiological differences between men and women. Add to that personality differences, cultural differences, and differences in the way you were raised, and you may wonder how the two of you ever get along. The differences seem too numerous and insurmountable. Many women might throw up their hands in frustration, but as Christians we believe our differences can cause us to lift up our hands in praise. God's created differences between men and women are nothing short of holy. Differences bring balance, fullness, and completion to a marriage. We each have something to teach; we each have something to learn.

In the movie *Rocky,* the not-so-articulate boxer played by Sylvester Stallone made a profound observation about his girlfriend, Adrian. "She's got gaps; I got gaps. Together we fill gaps." Your husband fills your gaps. You fill his.

In summing up sexual differences, we suggest you think of women being like water and men being like ice cubes. Men and women are made from the same substance but are different in form. Men, like an ice cube, tend to be hard, fixed, and concentrated. Women, like water, are more lucid and flowing, whether in their relationships or in their verbal communication. Sexual intercourse between a husband and wife is much like putting an ice cube into a glass of water. The man comes into the woman, hard and separate from her, but as they linger in intimate touch, they melt together in oneness. The man loses his hard edge, the woman is filled up by him. As they melt together in sexual love, differences dissolve.

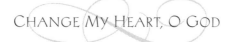

CHANGE MY HEART, O GOD

1. Read this chapter together with your husband. As you read, pause to talk about any statements that ring true in your marriage. Then take turns completing the following statements:

    ~& Three things I appreciate about you that are different from me are (fill in the blank).
    ~& Three things I enjoy doing with you are (fill in blank).
    ~& When it comes to sex, I really like it when you (fill in blank).
    ~& One thing new I'd like to try sexually is (fill in blank).

2. Reread the difference dissolvers on pages 37-41 and choose one to apply this week.

• you can look at things analytically
• you are good at financial things
• you are a good teacher
• going on vacations
• driving in the car
  going on walks

• are very gentle

⚮

DIFFERENCES IN SEXUALITY

	Men	Women
Orientation	Physical	Relational
	Compartmentalized	Wholistic
	Physical oneness	Emotional oneness
	Variety	Security
	Sex is high priority	Other priorities may be higher
Stimulation	Sight	Touch
	Smell	Attitudes
	Body-centered	Actions
		Words
		Person-centered
Needs	Respect	Understanding
	Admiration	Love
	Physically needed	Emotionally needed
	Not to be put down	Time
Sexual Response	Acyclical	Cyclical
	Quick excitement	Slow excitement
	Initiates (usually)	Responder (usually)
	Difficult to distract	Easily distracted
Orgasm	Propagation of species	Propagation of oneness
	Shorter, more intense	Longer, more in-depth
	Physically oriented	Emotionally oriented
	Orgasm usually needed for satisfaction	Satisfaction possible without orgasm

These are general tendencies and are not true in all cases.[12]

What Do I Do When I Don't Want to Do It?

A scene from a movie shows a husband and wife each talking with their therapists. On the left half of a split screen, the man complains, "We *hardly ever* have sex. Maybe three times a week, tops." On the right half of the screen the woman laments, "We are *constantly* having sex. We must have it two or three times a week!"

In the movie, this was meant to be a humorous scene, but it's not funny if the dialog hits home. Can you identify with this woman? In your mind, is sex with your husband a BIG issue—he wants more, you want less? If so, ask yourself how much time you think you and your husband will spend making love during your lifetime. How many hours this month? This week?

According to Dr. Ed Wheat, author of *Intended for Pleasure*, the average couple spends no more than one hour a week in lovemaking. Does this surprise you? When a woman feels stretched beyond her limit with trying to balance all her roles in life, lovemaking can become just one more thing to check off her list.

If you are struggling with "not wanting to do it," we encourage you to ask yourself why. Is it because you are overwhelmed with life, and sex just isn't as important as the other fifty items on your list? Are you hurt or angry over something your husband did and you don't want to be physically close to him? Do you have a tainted view of sex? Have you allowed yourself to have incorrect thought patterns?

If your lack of interest sexually is the result of problems in your marriage, we urge you to seek professional help from a pastor or a Christian counselor. But for many women, the problem is not their marriage, it's their attitude. They don't want to "do it" because they have not made a commitment to God to be the lover He has asked them to be. In this chapter, we want to address attitude.

First, let's define the word. Attitude is an inward feeling expressed by outward behavior. Perhaps you think your husband isn't aware of your attitude. Believe us—he knows. What you are inside shows itself in your facial expressions, tone of voice, and body language. You may not say the words, but every part of you shouts, "I don't want to do this!"

Look at these three attitudes wives have about sex, and honestly ask yourself, "Which attitude best describes me?"

- "Sex is something I do because I have to."
- "Sex is something I do because God says I have to."
- "Sex is a way I can give love to my husband and minister to him."

Perhaps your attitude is a bit more . . . blunt!

- "Sex is a thankless chore."
- "The best thing about sex is when it's over."
- "I've got better things to do, but once again I crawl between the sheets so my husband can have his jollies."
- "Sex isn't important to me, and I really don't care about making it a priority."
- "Sex requires too much effort."
- "What *is* my husband's problem? Did he get a triple dose of testosterone in the womb? For once, can't he leave me alone?"

What Is God's Attitude?

Let's compare our attitudes to the attitude God wants us to have. Look with us at a familiar passage, one that has been very misunderstood. It's the portion of the Bible that some women interpret to mean they have to perform their "wifely duty."

> Let the husband fulfill his duty to his wife, and likewise also the wife
> to her husband. The wife does not have authority over her own body,

but the husband does; and likewise also the husband does not have authority over his own body, but the wife does. Stop depriving one another, except by agreement for a time that you may devote yourselves to prayer, and come together again lest Satan tempt you because of your lack of self-control. (1 Corinthians 7:3-5)

Do we hear you saying, "But it *does* say the wife has a duty to meet the sexual needs of her husband"? Before you put this chapter down, please be willing to listen with an open heart to what the passage is really saying.

The word *duty* in English carries with it the idea of an unpleasant task. But the message conveyed by the Greek word is that "of a debt." It is not the conferring of a favor ("Okay, I'll accommodate you") but the payment of a debt that is owed. Three important principles are embedded in this passage: the principle of need, the principle of authority, and the principle of faithfulness. As we look at these principles, you will see that husband and wife have not only the freedom but also the responsibility to please the other sexually and to be pleased in return.

1. The principle of need. God gave us the gift of sexual need (verse 3). God's Word commands—it does not suggest—that we meet our mate's sexual needs because we both have these needs. Sexual passion is a God-given gift. You may not view it as a gift, but just as good health and children are gifts from God, so is our ability to be one with our husbands through a physical union. When we grasp hold of this and begin to do all we can to meet our husband's need, the relationship will be blessed with intimate oneness and physical pleasure.

2. The principle of authority. When we marry, we actually participate in a gift exchange (verse 4). The wife gives the gift of her body to her husband, and he gives the gift of his body to her. Each gives up the right to his or her own body and turns that authority over to the other. This is an awesome concept. Sadly, we quickly learn that one of the easiest ways to hurt our mate is to withhold the gift of our bodies. But God makes it clear that we do not have this right.

3. The principle of faithfulness. Verse 5 contains strong language, warning us not to take back the gift of our body given on our wedding day. God has said that with the gift comes a privileged responsibility to allow the other to enjoy the gift. We're told, "Stop depriving one another." The text literally says, "Do not commit fraud by taking back what has been pledged."

The only reason Scripture gives for abstaining from frequent sexual encounters is prayer. We've heard a myriad of reasons why women don't want to have sex, but prayer is not on their lists. According to this verse, if we refuse to make love for other reasons, we open our marriage to satanic temptations. As has been said, the Creator who gave us our sexual desire knows this, so He instructs us to participate actively and regularly in sex with our mate. Biblically, sex is not a debatable issue. It is an integral part of marriage.

In *The Message*, verse 4 is paraphrased: "Marriage is a decision to serve the other, whether in bed or out." Because God gave us the gift of sex, and we gave our individual bodies as gifts to our husbands, we are indebted to each other. Sex is not an unpleasant duty but a privileged responsibility. Sexual relations between a husband and wife are God-ordained and commanded. Failure of either to yield sexually to the authority of their spouse brings dishonor to God because it dishonors marriage.

ATTITUDE IS EVERYTHING

Some of you may be thinking, Linda and Lorraine, is Scripture saying I can never say "not tonight?" No, but we would caution you to be very careful about how you say it. Men are very vulnerable in the sexual area. You may think women are sensitive in this area, but men are even more sensitive. Remember, their feelings about their masculinity are wrapped up in their prowess as a lover. Your husband feels emotionally rejected when you turn down his sexual advances. It is important that wives understand the vulnerability a man has in offering himself to her.

If you just can't make love right when he asks, here are some suggested responses:

> "Honey, I love you, and I want to make love to you later. Right now I'm
> so tense from being with the kids (or at work) all day that I wouldn't be
> able to love you the way I want to. Please just hold me for a minute. If

you would help me with the kids, we can plan some time after they're in bed."

"I've rarely said no in the past, I'm not saying no for the future, I'm just saying no for this moment."

"Honey, I am literally too tired to respond. Please let me just give love to you. That gives me so much pleasure."

Yes, there are ways to lovingly say "later" or "for now, let me satisfy you," but we must remember that God says we are to give our bodies as a gift. Perhaps you think that since we are writing a book on sex, both of us are always ready and eager to make love. Not so. Like you, we get tired. We have wacko hormones. We often have "more important" things on our minds. Sometimes we find ourselves irritated with our husbands and don't want to be in the same room with them, let alone the same bed. But we've made a commitment to honor God and be exciting lovers to our husbands. That decision helps our attitudes when sex is the last thing on our minds.

Our friend Brooke told us that she recently struggled with her attitude, yet made the choice to honor her commitment to her husband. She shares the following story from her journal:

> Driving home on the snowy roads, my heart was singing. Tonight I would be alone. Jake had a basketball game with the church league and the children were each invited to a sleepover. An empty house. What joy! Visions of slipping into a bubble bath with a good book and a cup of hot chocolate danced in my mind.
>
> When the garage door opened, I saw our blue car. Jake was still home. I was totally unprepared for him and his plan for the evening. With a grin, he informed me that a night of lovemaking awaited me in front of the fire. My heart sunk to my feet. I was anticipating alone-ness—not togetherness.
>
> I felt sad that my evening alone had vanished. Sex was the last thing on my mind. Perhaps I could get up for hors d'oeuvre sex, but it was obvious Jake wanted Thanksgiving dinner with all the trimmings! I just wasn't in the mood. What was I to do?

My thoughts went to a conversation I'd had with a friend. She told me her husband never wanted her. I should be grateful that after seventeen years of marriage, Jake still yearned for me, that he preferred a romantic evening with me over a basketball game. But I wasn't. Not tonight. *Help, God,* I prayed. *I love this man. Help me want to love him.* One decision followed another. I prayed that Jake would not see how hard this was for me.

I told Jake how much I loved him, told him how I was going to give him pleasure, but my mind and heart were in the bath with my book. I continued to pray and love my husband. *I choose to love him, Lord. Give me desire for him.*

As I write, it's hours later. My Jake is asleep. I can't sleep because I'm still thinking about what happened tonight. It was a beautiful time of lovemaking—exquisite. Afterward we felt so close and intimate.

What a lesson for me. Yes, my plan was shattered, but how grateful I am that I made a choice and went with the new plan. I made one husband very happy, and I'm at peace that I chose to love. And someday, God will even have an evening alone for me.

Brooke had to make some hard choices to change her attitude but what a difference it made. She chose to give unselfishly and to allow God to work.

LET GOD WORK

We don't know the number of sexual relationships sabotaged by a wife's poor attitude, but we know it is high. When it comes to sex, we must each answer the question: Will I selfishly demand to have my own way, or will I minister to my husband and trust that God will bless my obedience?

Imagine this scene. It's evening. Your husband splashes on Polo and crawls into bed. *Oh no!* you think. *Not tonight.* Outwardly you are calm, but a vicious game of tug of war rages within. *I don't want to do it!* your selfish nature yanks. *By God's grace, I will do it,* your loving nature tugs. Your husband snuggles closer. His hand caresses your thigh. Your mind and emotions battle. *I won't! I will!* Which voice wins?

In moments like these, we ask God to strike us with a severe case of the "willies."

I WILL deny my selfishness and respond to my husband.

I WILL give my body as a gift.

I WILL enjoy sex and praise God for creating this beautiful way to relate to my husband.

I WILL minister to my husband and think of his needs rather than my own.

Making the right decision is never easy but there are benefits to adopting the right attitude. When we choose to love selflessly, we honor God, we make our husbands happy, and we find more pleasure in our lovemaking.

Dying to self is difficult, but it is necessary if you want to grow in godliness. Being godly means having a godly attitude. Godly attitudes result in godly actions, such as giving your body to your husband. This is easier if you surrender to God and allow His Spirit to work within you. "Nothing is impossible with God" (Luke 1:37, NIV). He is able to give you desire where none existed before. He can help you exchange wrong thinking with godly thinking. He can cause you to enjoy deeper intimacy than you ever thought possible.

> *God, I confess that I have not always appreciated Your gift of sex— or even wanted it. I have shunned You and withheld my body from my husband. Forgive me. I want to be a willing and creative lover— but it's hard. Please stir up in me passion and desire for my husband. Help me get my mind off myself and focus instead on him. I surrender myself to You and humbly ask that You begin now to work in me.*

CHANGE MY HEART, O GOD

We have defined attitude as an inward feeling expressed by outward behavior. What happens in our minds will soon display itself in our actions. If we adopt God's viewpoint about sex, if we transform our minds and yield to His attitude, the inward choices will blossom into loving actions with our husband.

1. Take a few minutes and ask yourself the following questions:

   - What is my sexual attitude?
   - How would I rate my attitude? Excellent, good, fair, poor, or lousy?
   - In what way would God desire my attitude to change?

2. Next, do the following short projects:

   - Write a personal paraphrase of 1 Corinthians 7:3-5.
   - Determine one creative thing you can do this week to live 1 Corinthians 7:3-5.

FOUR WAYS TO JUMP-START YOUR SEXUAL DESIRE

1. Try a tad of testosterone. We often associate testosterone with males, but females also produce this hormone throughout their lives, only in reduced levels. "Testosterone acts on the brain to stimulate sexual interest and may also affect sensitivity to sexual stimulation and orgasmic ability in both sexes."[1] Circumstances that may warrant additional testosterone include a marked decrease in sexual desire, menopause, and drop in ovarian function.

Zinc is critical to the production of testosterone in both women and men.[2] Foods rich in zinc are oysters and pumpkin seeds. Make oyster stew, sprinkle pumpkin seeds on your salad, or take zinc tablets. If the natural approaches fail, ask your physician if a tad of testosterone would lift your libido.

2. Exercise your "desire" muscle. Shift into sexual gear by exercising the PC (pubococcygeal muscle). (See chapter 16, pages 191-2 for more information and instructions on how to exercise your desire muscle.)

3. Exercise your body. Energy is essential to feeling sexual. Sedentary bodies and overstuffed stomachs are energy robbers. Who wants to make love when they're so full, they can't budge their bulge? One woman said, "I enjoy making love on an empty stomach but when I'm full, forget it." Just as an empty tummy can make you hungry for sex, so can exercise. Research shows that the sexual appetite of women who had exercised soared in comparison with those who hadn't. Increased heart rate and breathing mimics the signs of arousal, jump-starting the body for sexual stimulation. In addition, it's been proven that exercise increases testosterone levels.[3]

4. Natural aphrodisiacs. Both kava and saw palmetto have a long tradition as aphrodisiacs and can be found in capsule and liquid form in health-food stores. Damiana, a shrub indigenous to the Southwest and the Mexican desert, has been used by the people of this region as an aphrodisiac. (See chapter 11, page 130 for additional information.) Without a doubt, the very best aphrodisiac can't be bought at a health-food store, nor does it grow in the Amazon; but it is always at your disposal. It is your brain. Remember, your mind *is* your most important sexual organ. (See chapter 3, "How Do I Shift into Sexual Gear?")

six

Where Can I Go to Buy a New Body?

*W*e asked twenty-five friends, "Are you satisfied with your body?" They all said no.

Few women are pleased with their bodies. Many complain that they are too tall, too short, too thin, or too prone to gain weight. Others say their hair is too curly or too straight. There are those who hate their noses, christening them too big, too long, or too "pugged." And how many women yearn for bigger breasts, the symbol in American society of "sexy"? Many, if cosmetic surgeons are to be believed.

We look in the mirror and cringe, then look at someone else and think, *If I had a body like that, I'd be satisfied.* Think again. Actress Julia Roberts has a body to die for, yet she had a stand-in for the nude scenes in *Pretty Woman* because her body wasn't "good enough."[1] Meg Ryan has an enviable body punctuated with an adorable smile. But Meg says of herself, "I think I'm kind of weird looking. If I could change the way I look, I'd like to have longer legs, smaller feet, a smaller nose . . ."[2]

Why are we so critical of our bodies? One reason is because the media constantly bombards us with messages designed to produce body dissatisfaction. Svelte models endorsing fat-free delights or exercise equipment suggest our bodies will never look good unless we buy their products. Merchandisers imply that if we want a beautiful body, we must purchase this bust-enhancing bra or that torso-lengthening swimsuit. Magazine articles add to our body discomfort with headlines like, "Lose Ten Pounds in Ten Days" or "Learn Beauty Secrets to Help You Look like the Supermodels."

Another reason women are dissatisfied with their bodies is society's constantly changing beauty standards. In the Renaissance, round and rotund was the ideal. In the sixties, the perfect body was a Marilyn Monroe prototype: average height, blond, buxom, and curvy. Ten years later, curvy Marilyn was out, and tall, pencil-thin Twiggy was in. With such shifting standards, what's a body to do?

A third reason is that the current beauty standards are impossible to achieve. As we near the twenty-first century, the rules for a beautiful body are

Thou shalt not age.

Thou shalt be thin.

Thou shalt have perfectly symmetrical, large, firm breasts.[3]

The standard is "Thou shalt not age," but we *will* age. The second law of thermodynamics states that everything moves downhill to a more disorderly state. After age forty, we've discovered, the speed of deterioration rivals records set at the Indianapolis 500! An article called "How Old Is Your Body?" reports this delightful tidbit: "Around age thirty, muscle mass slowly begins to decline and is replaced by slow-burning fat."[4]

The standard is "Thou shalt be thin," but we *will* gain weight. Women with hourglass figures often discover that their sand slides toward the bottom with the passage of time. Weight gain is a growing problem (pun intended). In 1984, 56 percent of adults over age twenty-five said they were heavier than the recommended weight for their body type. In 1998, this figure rose to 76 percent.[5] One article we read said the body "automatically gains one pound each year after age forty."[6] (Both of our bodies substantiate this statistic!)

The standard is "Thou shalt have perfectly symmetrical large, firm, breasts," but not all our breasts are large, and our breasts will sag. Romans 8:20 says creation is subjected to futility. In essence, creation is sagging; this includes our personal creation—skin, muscles, even our once perky breasts.

As long as we continue to listen to the world's messages about our bodies, we will never be satisfied with how we look. Let's face it. There are three billion women in the world who don't look like the supermodels and only seven who do. Instead of listening to the world's message, we need to listen to what God says. God's message is: *"Rejoice in the body I gave you. Use it to honor Me and please your husband."*

THE VIEW IN GOD'S MIRROR

> I will give thanks to Thee, for I am fearfully and wonderfully made; wonderful are Thy works, and my soul knows it very well. (Psalm 139:14)

I (Lorraine) desire to see myself through God's eyes, but I wrestle with a worldly mind-set. Several years ago, I was disgusted with myself because I'd put on weight and my clothes were uncomfortably tight. I couldn't stand the thought of Peter touching my newly formed cellulite, and I side-stepped his attempts to be intimate. One night, in a moment of honesty, I admitted: "I don't feel sexy. I just feel fat." The roll around my stomach didn't bother Peter, but he realized it greatly inhibited me. He said, "Honey, your thinking about your body is wrong. I have an idea to help you. I am going to write Psalm 139:14 on a sheet of paper. I want you to tape this to the bathroom mirror, then stand in front of the mirror naked for a half-hour. Review each part of your body from the head down, and thank God that you are fearfully and wonderfully made."

Looking at myself naked was not my idea of fun (in my present state it was nothing short of frightening) but never being one to resist a challenge, I locked the bathroom door and shed my clothes.

Immediately my eyes went to the thickness around my waist, but I had promised Peter I would start with the top of my body and work my way down. I touched my hair. It is one of my best features. *Thank you, God, for blessing me with such thick hair. I am fearfully and wonderfully made,* I prayed. I studied my face. True, there were more wrinkles than last year, but some of the tiny ones around my eyes had come from laughing. I had always liked my blue eyes. I marveled at the incredible gift of sight these two round objects afforded me. I closed my eyes in a prayer of conviction, *Forgive me, God, for taking my sight for granted.* When I opened them, again, I saw my body with new eyes. How creative God was! How did He think to put graceful feathery lashes at the edge of the eyelid? How interestingly He fashioned our noses to separate the eyes, and to act as a funnel for enjoying smells. I studied my ears, my teeth, my mouth, and tongue. *Oh God, I AM fearfully and wonderfully made.*

I stayed in the bathroom a long time, praising God for the remarkable weaving together of the body. I stroked the muscles in my arms, examined the joints and veins in my hands, praised God for His wisdom in choosing four fingers and a thumb to enable me to grasp objects. I touched my breasts and praised God for flowing sustenance from them to my children. I rubbed my hand over my not-so-flat stomach, but just below the stomach felt the scar from the C-section of my first child. The stretch marks and extra inch around the waist were worthwhile exchanges for the two children that graced our home. I went over my body, then kneeled in praise: "God, forgive me. I've been focusing on all the wrong things. I've obsessed about trivia, when my body has been personally fashioned by You. I give thanks to You. Wonderful are Your works, for I am fearfully and wonderfully made."

God desires that we praise Him for the gift of our bodies, and that we accept who He created us to be. The message God sends about our bodies is *"Rejoice in the body I gave you. Use it to honor Me and to please your husband."*

THE BEAUTY OF A SENSUOUS WOMAN

It is difficult to use our bodies to please our husbands when we don't feel attractive or sexy. Let's take a look at these two words and see how they relate to being a sensuous lover.

What does it mean to be attractive? Webster defines attractive as "having the quality of attracting; having the power of charming or alluring; inviting; engaging, enticing." But it is difficult to feel attractive when we are obsessing

WHAT DO MEN LOOK AT?

What do you think men look at first when they see a woman? If you answer "her body," you are wrong. According to a *USA Today* survey, 39 percent of men say the first thing they notice are eyes. Next highest (25 percent) is smile or teeth. Only 14 percent say the first thing they notice is the body.[7]

What kind of body do you think attracts men? Do you think men prefer the lithe supermodel look? No. The average man finds normal-weight women sexier than very thin women. This was the conclusion of Dr. Devendra Singh, University of Texas psychologist, after showing pictures of twelve female shapes to seven hundred men.[8]

about a new roll of fat or our size double A breasts. We try to laugh it off: "I'm so flat you could land airplanes on my chest" or "My legs look like tree stumps." But such degrading comments can sabotage our body image and cause us to feel unattractive when we are naked in the bedroom. We'd feel more attractive if our bodies looked a certain way, if we had a perfect "10" body. But Dr. John Gray, author of *Mars and Venus in the Bedroom*, says, "When a man is in love and turned on by his wife, he is also totally entranced by the feminine beauty of her body, regardless of where the media would rank it on a scale of one to ten. When he is in love with his wife, he experiences the perfection of her body for him."[9]

The issue for you personally is what is attractive to your husband? Most men prefer women who are average weight but some men like women who are overweight. Others like the hard body type. Some men like women with the glamour image and lots of makeup. Others prefer the natural look. Rather than seeking to please fashion critics, we should seek to please the man God gave us to love.

Your body, along with everything else that makes up you, attracted your husband to you. You allured him, captured him with your smile, eyes, body, intelligence, personality, all of you. Out of all the women in the world, he chose you. It wasn't just your body he liked, it was you. It doesn't matter if you are 4'11" and short-waisted, or 5'11" with long legs. If you do the most with what you have, your body will turn your husband on.

Let's take a look at the second word, *sexy*. According to Andrew Greeley, author of *Sexual Intimacy*, to be sexy is to be aware of your body as an instrument of playfulness and delight, to be able to communicate this awareness to your husband and give him the gift of your body for pleasure, delight, variety, and playfulness.[10]

We're going to tell you a secret. It's better to be sensuous than to have a perfect "10" body. Delighting your husband with your breasts and giving him ecstasy (Proverbs 5:19), swaying your hips seductively and displaying your body before him (Song of Solomon 6:13–7:9) will cause him to revel in the joy of your body. It is God's gift to him. Your body is for him!

Our bodies are far from perfect. And they will continue to age, but we can learn to be experts at using them to intoxicate our husbands with delight. Listen and learn from Carolyn, a wise wife who will soon be sixty.

> As I age, the old body deteriorates. I've got stretch marks from three babies, cellulite, and varicose veins. My breasts sag, wrinkles abound, but as my body has fallen, my expertise as a lover has risen. I really think my dear husband of forty years still sees my body as it was when I was young because he receives such pleasure from it.

Carolyn knew that nothing is as "sexy" as a woman who gives in to her sensuousness, a woman who enjoys sex and lets her husband know she loves to give and receive pleasure. Consider the following statement: "Nothing transcends the traditional definitions of beauty like the face and body of a passionately aroused woman."[11]

The message God gives is good: *"Rejoice in the body I gave you. Use it to honor Me and please your husband."*

TAKING CARE OF THE BODY GOD GAVE ME

No mail-order catalogue sells new bodies. Until we get our heavenly body, the one we have is it. And really, when you think about it, the body you currently have is remarkable. Not only is it capable of great sensuous pleasure but, for a Christian, it is also the place of residence for the living God.

> Do you not know that your body is a temple of the Holy Spirit, who is in you, whom you have received from God? You are not your own; you were bought at a price. Therefore honor God with your body. (1 Corinthians 6:19-20, NIV)

Have you ever meditated on this verse? Imagine. God chose your body to be the home where His Spirit lives. Webster defines a temple as a "consecrated place . . . a place dedicated to the service or worship of God." These thoughts inspire us to make our temples as fit and as lovely as possible.

At times, both of us have been tempted to give up the battle against the bulge and our commitment to healthy eating and exercise. Gravity is winning so why keep fighting? Two reasons: First we want to glorify God in our bodies—to be a "fit temple" for God to dwell in, and second, we want to be creative, sensuous, playful lovers to our husbands.

So we determine to fight the fight. We apply our hearts to discipline (Proverbs 23:12). We buffet our bodies so we will not be enslaved to their appetites (1 Corinthians 9:27). We persevere so we will not become what Scripture calls a sluggard.

The sluggard is mentioned thirteen times in the book of Proverbs, and in each instance, the warning is "Don't be lazy and undisciplined" (Proverbs 6:6-11; 24:30-34; 26:13-16). This lazy woman is described as turning on her bed like a door turns on its hinges (Proverbs 26:14). The simile points to her immobility. She will not take action. She turns over and over in her bed without making any progress toward rising. When we talk and complain about how we need to eat right and exercise, saying, "I'm disgusted with myself. I should join a gym" or "I'd diet, except Christmas is coming," we are like the sluggard. We make excuses and procrastinate.

Procrastination is a professional thief whose specialty is stealing. He does not plunder jewels but rather motivation and incentive. He steals our love of ourselves as sensuous women. He steals the possibilities of joy and freedom for us and our husbands. Do you know this thief? We do. We have stepped on the bathroom scale and shrieked, "I simply can't weigh that much." We have been known to remove several articles of clothing and our earrings—even all but one contact lens—so we can see the numbers on the scale. Mercilessly, the dial tells the truth. But the thief of procrastination offers another interpretation: "You're just bloated. The scale is wrong." Snatching our surge of motivation, he whispers the magic word, *mañana,* and we reach for the bag of Doritos.[12]

None of us likes to admit our lack of discipline, but we must face it. If we are overweight and sedentary, it affects our physical health, our energy level, the way we feel about ourselves, and our sexuality. We need to replace the word *mañana* with the one word which shoos away procrastination: NOW.

Not only does the lazy woman make excuses instead of taking action, she will not finish things. Both of us are skilled starters. When we begin a diet program, such commitment is rarely seen. But after a week of eating rabbit food, our motivation fizzles out. (There is just no comfort in carrots.)

The two of us live a few miles from each other. Last year, we held one another accountable as we embarked on a vigorous exercise-and-eat-right program. After months of hard work, we each went down a size. I (Linda) raced to a seamstress to have a skirt altered. What fun to watch her pull in the seams and make it smaller. How disappointing to return to that same seamstress ten months later and have her let out the same skirt. Statistics indicate 95 percent of the people who lose weight regain it all in five years.[13] We both wound up a statistic. Even still, we are determined not to give up, and we remind ourselves of the reasons we need to persevere.

LEARN FROM WHAT YOU SEE

The wise woman observes the lazy person and reflects:

> I passed by the field of the [lazy woman], and by the vineyard of the [woman] lacking sense; and behold, it was completely overgrown with thistles, its surface was covered with nettles, and its stone wall was broken down. When I saw, I reflected upon it; I looked, and received instruction. (Proverbs 24:30-32)

If we apply this to our discussion of our bodies, it would read something like this.

> A wise woman visited a friend she had not seen for years and was shocked by the changes. Once an attractive and vibrant woman, her friend had neglected her "vineyard." It was overgrown and ungroomed. The wise woman observed her friend's depressed countenance and lack of energy and learned from what she saw.

Do we learn from what we see in ourselves and in others? We are in the process of learning—and it *is* a process. As we've talked with other women about body discipline, and as we've battled with being lazy ourselves, we've found help in this advice.

1. Get God's perspective. God's Word is a mirror. When we look into it, we see a reflection. Have you ever walked through a carnival fun house and looked in one mirror that made you look like a string bean, another that made you look like an elephant, and yet another that distorted your shape into an alien form? When we view our bodies through the world's standard of ever-youthful, thin, and busty, we see a distorted image. But when we hold up the mirror of Scripture and see God's standard, we see clearly. We are "fearfully and wonderfully made."

2. Don't beat yourself up. The goal is not to be a certain size or shape. The goal is to do the most with what you have and only put things in your body that benefit your "temple." We know women who have nice figures but who throw junk food in their bodies and haven't exercised since their high-school gym class. We know other women who diligently work out every day and eat only organic salads but can't get the scale to move down. If you are being faithful to take care of your body, give yourself grace.

3. Make the most of what God gave you. Because we are made in God's image, there is no such thing as an ugly woman, only a woman who fails to take care of herself. Ask your hairdresser what hairstyle is best suited for you. Schedule a makeover at a department store, and discover something to give you a new look. Find a color consultant and learn what colors enhance your skin tone and which clothing styles compliment your body. We both have blond hair (thanks to a bottle) and blue eyes, but the orange that makes Lorraine glow makes Linda look like she has the flu, and the hot pink that makes Linda sparkle makes Lorraine look washed out. There is much we can do immediately to make us look and feel better about ourselves.

4. Enlist the help of others. Goals are easier in groups. Success is multiplied when you do it with someone else. When I (Linda) lived in Hong Kong, I got together with friends to form a diet club, complete with theme song and reward system. Accountability can help you persevere through the difficult times and make the discipline process fun. Excellent gyms and wonderful weight-reduction programs are available. We highly recommend the biblically based program, Weigh Down Workshop.[14]

5. Be realistic. Neither of us has a body type that works in a size six or eight. We would kill ourselves achieving and trying to maintain a six because that is not who we are. A more realistic goal for us is to lose ten pounds, firm up what we have, and keep firming it up. What's a realistic goal for you?

FINDING THE BALANCE

God instructs us to be disciplined. He also says we are fearfully and wonderfully made and tells us we are to accept the body He gave us. The key
word is balance. Some women go overboard on the grace and acceptance;
"God loves me like I am." Other women go overboard on the law and discipline, obsessing over their bodies to the point it becomes sin. It is a constant struggle to balance the two, but we must if we are going to adhere
to God's message: *"Rejoice in the body I gave you. Use it to honor Me and to
please your husband."*

When you begin to see the balance between accepting the way God
made you and being responsible for your body, you can become free to be
the sensuous and exciting lover God desires you to be, free to concentrate
on giving and receiving pleasure rather than on what you look like.

According to a survey from *Psychology Today*, one of the quickest and
best ways to feel good about your body is to have a rewarding sexual relationship with your husband. Good sexual experiences breed high levels of
body satisfaction.[15] It's a circle. When you feel good about your body, you
can be an exciting lover, and when you have a wonderfully free sexual relationship in your marriage, you feel better about your body.

There is no place to go to buy a new body. Each wife can grow to be
attractive and sexy. There is a natural beauty that emanates from a woman
who has done the most with what she has and has learned to use her body
to delight and entice her husband.

Will you ask God to search your heart?

> *God, what are you saying to me? Do I need to accept the body You
> gave me, develop the beauty of a sensuous wife, or be more respon-
> sible with my "temple"? Lord, show me what You want. I desire to
> rejoice in the body You gave me and use it to honor You and please
> my husband.*

CHANGE MY HEART, O GOD

1. Write out Psalm 139:14 on a sheet of paper and tape it to your mirror. Then stand naked in front of the bathroom mirror. Review your body from the top down and praise God for how "fearfully and wonderfully" you are made.

2. Write a paragraph describing how you can use your body to delight and intoxicate your husband.

3. Read about the lazy person in Proverbs 6:6-11; 24:30-34; 26:13-16 and ask if any of these descriptions apply to you. What will you begin this week? Determine one step you can take to better care for your "temple" (limit candy bars to once a month, exercise five minutes more each day, have a makeover at a department store).

4. On a scale of one to ten, how much focus do you place on your body, with one being no focus and ten being obsessed? What can you do to bring more balance to this area of your life?

FACTS ABOUT SEX THAT MAY SURPRISE YOU

- Sex is good exercise. Every time you make love you burn between 100 and 150 calories. That's as many calories as you'll burn in a brisk twenty-minute walk![16]

- Sex is good medicine. Studies indicate that women's pain thresholds rise during sexual activity. This means chronic conditions like arthritis, low-back pain, and even PMS may be helped.[17]

- Sex improves skin tone and color by increasing blood flow and helping skin to regenerate and become more pliable and elastic.[18]

- Sex stimulates endorphin release, which enables you to sleep more soundly.[19]

- Sex is a great cardiovascular workout. During sex, the heart rate may reach 130 beats a minute.[20]

seven

How Do I Make Love with Children Wrapped Around My Knees?

*M*y gynecologist told me six weeks after Kelsey was born that I could resume normal sexual relations with my husband," said Beth, a twenty-eight-year-old first-time mom. "What a joke! Since the birth of my daughter, nothing in my life is normal, especially sex."

From the moment she first cuddled Kelsey in her arms, Beth's world changed. She loved the new sensations that greeted her—when she could comprehend them through the fog of exhaustion. Weary and sleep-deprived, Beth ranked her enthusiasm for sex right up there with mopping the floor. Even if she did desire to be intimate with her husband, where could she find the time and energy to enjoy it? Beth looked forward to the day when life would return to normal.

Like Beth, many new moms believe life will return to normal, "*after* I recover from my episiotomy, *after* my hormones quit ricocheting like a pin-ball machine, *after* the 3 A.M. feedings end, *after* I lose these extra twenty pounds." The problem with this thinking is that once you have kids, normal is a misnomer. You are changed. Your husband is changed. Your home environment is changed. Your love life will change too.

According to a survey of almost six thousand parents by *Parenting* magazine, 80 percent of husbands and wives agree that their sex life had suffered as a result of having children. We wish we could spin around like Wonder Woman and instantly transform from maternal mother to sexy lover and back again. But when the kids are crying at the same time our husbands are sighing, this seems impossible. In our new role as mothers, sometimes sleep sounds better than sex. That was certainly the case for both of us.

DENTED CANS OF PEAS AND ZOMBIES

Lorraine

Caring for two needy toddlers drained the life out of me. I often felt like a lazy Susan spinning round and round with my children constantly pulling boxes and cans off my shelf. The baby needed to be fed, bathed, and changed. Caring for her needs was like pulling boxes of cereal off my shelf. My three-year-old and I argued about what she should wear. Getting her dressed was like pulling crackers off my shelf. Amanda fell down the stairs; Megan bumped her head on the crib. Doctoring their "owies" emptied my shelf of juice. At 11 P.M., I'd collapse into bed, dizzy, empty, and exhausted, and then Peter would snuggle up next to me.

One night he pulled me close, and I muttered, "Oh no! All I have left is a can of dented peas." Certain he had heard me incorrectly, he asked, "What did you say?" Suddenly I remembered a decision I had made years ago to always be available for my husband. Tired as I was, I WOULD be there for him. So I changed my comment from "Oh no, all I have left is a can of dented peas," to "Okay. But do you mind if I don't move, please?"

Linda

I had three children within thirty-eight months and was tempted to change my name from Linda to Zombie. Jody sent me to a doctor to find out why I was so exhausted. What was not obvious to Jody was apparent to the doctor. "Linda, anyone with three children the ages of yours would be struggling to stay awake."

I felt as though my sexual desire had fallen asleep too. I knew I couldn't put my sexual relationship on hold until after the kids were grown, so I prayed, "Help, Lord! Show me how to get my mind back into sexual gear even now when I am numb from constant tiredness." I began to write T. S. on my calendar every other day. When Jody saw my calendar, he wondered who T. S. was and why I was spending so much time with this person. Years later he laughed when he learned T. S. was an abbreviation for

THINK SEX, my simple yet effective reminder to keep our sexual relationship a priority.

BEAT THE ODDS

Murphy's Law says: Sex makes little kids and kids make little sex. In one study, over six thousand couples were interviewed when they had no children and again five years later after they had become parents. The findings showed that after becoming parents, couples expressed a significant drop in marital satisfaction.[1] It's true, the years of rearing young kids can be one of the toughest times in a couple's marriage. But there is hope. A more encouraging survey discussed in *The Transition to Parenthood* says that of 250 couples surveyed, 20 percent experienced notable improvement in their marriages after having children.[2] This is the group to join! How can we improve the odds that we will be among the 20 percent who defied Murphy's Law? By making sex a priority.

Dr. Paul Pearsall, author of *Super Marital Sex*, writes: "Any part of the marriage that is ignored will disappear—particularly sex. For most couples, the amount of enjoyment they derive from their sexual relationship corresponds with the amount of attention they pay to it."[3] The truth is, if we don't make sex a priority when our children are three and five, we won't make sex a priority when they are thirteen and fifteen. We can't postpone lovemaking until the kids reach a better stage or there is nothing left on our to-do list.

Now is the time to act. We must pay attention. We do not have to live as though there is no tomorrow, but we had better love creatively as though there is only now.

Connie, a mother of seven (Did you get that? Seven!) said at a couples' retreat, "If you want to make sex a priority, you will find the time." By the glow on her husband's face and the number of car seats in her van, it was obvious that she not only found the time, she made the time.

Terri, mother of four children, wanted to make sex a priority but struggled to find the energy to do it. Here is how she solved her problem:

> I'm a morning person; my husband is a night owl. By the time he
> makes a move, I can't move because I'm too tired. But if I were

honest with myself, I'd admit that I can find a morsel of energy after the kids go down to diddle around the house, pick up, do laundry/dishes, etc. Because I am determined to make sex a priority, I choose to take that energy and channel it into the higher priority of showing the man of my life how I desire him. I do not wait for the mood, I just act. And for those times when I'm feeling hopelessly unenthused about lovemaking, I repeat the words of the Shulammite in Song of Solomon 5:16, "His mouth is most sweet. Yes, he is altogether lovely. He is my lover. He is my friend." Often these words arouse passion, but even if they don't, I still act because I know this is important.

Perhaps you are thinking, *Isn't it hypocritical to express love sexually when I'm not in the mood?* Gary Chapman, author of *The Five Love Languages*, has this response:

> Perhaps it would be helpful to distinguish between love as a feeling and love as an action. If you claim to have feelings that you do not have, that is hypocritical and such false communication is not the way to build intimate relationships. But if you express an act of love that is designed for the other person's benefit or pleasure, it is simply a choice. You are not claiming that the action grows out of a deep emotional bonding. You are simply choosing to do something for his benefit.[4]

Terri recently told us that she and her husband have a great sex life, a pretty amazing statement from a woman who has just had four babies in four and a half years. Terri is beating the odds and joining the 20 percent of couples who say marriage can be better *after* having kids. Though it was not easy, she chose to make sex a priority. Are you ready to make such a commitment? If so, we've got some practical ideas for you that might help.

CREATIVE HOME-COOKED SEX

To make sex a priority, you don't have to run out and buy a romantic getaway trip for two to Hawaii. With a little creativity, you can plan innovative excursions at home. The first matter of business is to establish your bedroom as your headquarters for lovemaking. (See chapter 19 for creating bedroom atmosphere.)

1. Reclaim your bedroom for sex. Liz and Samuel's bedroom had become the "gathering place," which was fine when thunder and lightning brought fears to little hearts. At first having the whole family under the covers felt cozy. Later on, it just felt crowded. Being kicked in the stomach by a pint-sized foot or knowing that at any moment a child would be in bed to snuggle put the kibosh on their sex life.

One morning over pancakes, they announced, "Kids, a new rule goes into effect today. No one is allowed in Mommy and Daddy's bedroom except Mommy and Daddy. Our bed is our private place where we go to talk. You have your private place in your own beds. We can all play and have fun together in any other part of the house, but our bedroom is off-limits."

If you feel Liz and Samuel went to extremes and you hate giving up cozy times in your bed, try restricting family gatherings in your bedroom to once a month. Or consider an alternative, like a family slumber party in the living room or a family read-a-thon in your kid's bedroom. Do what is comfortable for you, but make certain your children understand the need to respect your marriage bed as a sacred place set apart for the two of you.

2. Bedroom rendezvous. Now that your bedroom is your own again, plan a once-a-month bedroom extravaganza. Schedule the evening far in advance so you have time to plan and anticipate. Then take him to a place he's never been before . . . right in your bedroom! Create an exotic Caribbean ambiance by spreading two beach towels on the floor. Surround the towels with beach paraphernalia: beachballs, sunglasses, and bottles of coconut-scented suntan lotion. Whip up some tropical drinks, purchase a grass skirt and an "ocean sounds" tape, and aloha the evening away. Or transport your husband to a new place sexually by doing something you've never done before (see chapters 18 and 19 for ideas). The goal is to enhance your bedroom environment and to do something new in your lovemaking. Put all your creativity to work by planning something that will knock his socks off (and any other articles of clothing he may be wearing). Then have your husband plan next month's rendezvous with the challenge, "Can you top this?"

3. Home dates. Limited finances are never a reason to say no to dates. Reecie and Alex, who have four sons from six months to five years old, schedule dates at home. Once a month they swap childcare with another couple who is committed to keeping romance in their marriage. Their date lasts from about 4:30 P.M. to 8:00 P.M. Reecie explains how she pulls this off.

> I feed the kids and get them all jammied up so we can tuck them straight into bed after we pick them up. I also prepare dinner before Alex comes home—usually something simple—so cooking and clean up don't eat up our time together. We've had boxed macaroni by candlelight. What we eat is not the point (unless you're talking "dessert"—our name for treating ourselves to each other). And with the boys away, we can have "dessert" after dinner in any room of the house we choose!

Reecie says the hardest part about staying home for a date is the distractions. "I have to give myself a good talking to," she says. "I say, 'Reecie, this is not a time to play catch-up on household chores, but a time to concentrate on your lover.'"

4. Quickies on the menu. With three preschoolers in the house, Colleen and her husband were rarely having sex. "I decided we could at least have 'a quickie.' The kids were watching a video in the basement. I told Gene there was a leak in the upstairs bathroom that needed his attention. When he got to the door, I grabbed his hand, pulled him in, and turned the lock. We made love with me leaning against the sink. It was a little uncomfortable, but exhilarating! Now all I have to say is, 'Honey, there's a leak in the sink,' and he's upstairs in a flash!"

5. Saturday morning fun. Hire a babysitter to take the kids to the park for two hours while you and your husband enjoy time at home alone. Soak in a bubble bath together or give each other massages. It will be hard to decide who had more fun on this morning—the kids or you and your husband.

When you reclaim your bedroom for sex, when you bring back the quickie, when you schedule at-home dates and Saturday morning fun, you send the message to your husband: Loving you is a priority.

GET ME OUTTA HERE!

"There's no place like home" is a good theme song for lovemaking if we add a second chorus to the song: "There's no place like *away* from home." Extend the boundaries of physical passion beyond the walls of your home by regularly planning romantic getaways.

1. An anniversary escape. With little ones underfoot, getting away for a weekend may seem impossible, but even couples with caregiver restrictions and budget limitations can get away once a year for their anniversary. All it requires is a bit of advance planning.

I (Linda) recall one rainy anniversary when our children were small. Jody was speaking at a marriage conference at a local church. I was to join him and speak to the women that evening. My plan was to whisk him away after the conference to a lake cabin where we would spend a weekend alone. All day, I raced around packing suitcases, preparing special food to take, and writing instructions for the baby-sitter. Everything went wrong. I didn't feel good. The preparation took longer than I had planned. The children whined and said they didn't want me to go. As I drove across town in the rain, I cried and thought, *It's not worth all the effort. Why am I doing this anyway?*

After arriving at the conference, I spoke for three hours and was even more exhausted. I wished the suitcases weren't already in the car. I just wanted to go home and go to sleep. Jody and I walked to the car late that night and, opening the door, he saw the suitcases. "What are these for?" he asked. "Honey, I'm whisking you away to a lake cabin for a special anniversary surprise." The look on his face made my tiredness evaporate! I forgot all the tears and the hassle to get ready. Our two days were a time of basking in one other with NO responsibility! It was like a shot in the arm to our sexual relationship, and the fun and closeness stayed with us for weeks after returning home."

2. Triple trouble house swap. If you are thinking, *We could never get away alone; it's just not possible,* let us tell you about Kathleen. In less than two years, Kathleen had triplets and then another baby, giving her four children under two plus her five year old. (Don't you feel tired just reading about it?) The triplets were premature, and when they came home from the hospital, they came attached to oxygen tanks and heart monitors. Even still, a month later, Kathleen and Guy went away overnight to celebrate their anniversary. How did they arrange this? Nancy, a friend, came to Kathleen and Guy's house for the weekend and baby-sat their children while the weary parents went to Nancy's house and baby-sat her dogs. (Kathleen and Guy admit they got the better deal.) Did we mention that Nancy, in addition to being a loving and caring friend, was also a very capable registered nurse? Kathleen says, "Babies needs are important, but so is my marriage." If Kathleen can make a getaway a priority, so can we.

3. Adult time-outs. We send children to time-out to adjust their attitudes. Sometimes we need to send ourselves to "adult time-out" to adjust our attitudes. Schedule an adult time-out twice a month. Hire a baby-sitter, or if your budget is tight, arrange to "kid swap" with another couple. On your first time-out, go out to dinner someplace other than McDonald's. Look your best and wear your husband's favorite scent of perfume, instead of Eau de Baby Wipes. Slip into a silk blouse without any drool marks. Revel in the freedom of being able to walk into a restaurant carrying a classy purse instead of a bulky diaper bag. Plan to do something that's fun for both of you, but make sure you spend time looking into your husband's eyes and talking about something other than the children.

For your second time-out, consider having a motel date. (For specifics, read page 227.)

When you schedule adult time-outs, when you plan anniversary getaways, when you kid swap and house swap in order to be alone together, you send this message to your husband: Being with you is a priority.

Establish a caregiver network. You need baby-sitters who will watch your children for a few hours and for a few days. But if you don't have family nearby, where do you find them? Many YMCA programs and day-care centers offer baby-sitting training. Call and ask for the phone numbers of their top graduates. Check with your local high school and ask for names of reliable teenagers. Ask for recommendations from friends or people at your church. Sometimes preschool or elementary school teachers will baby-sit for extra cash. Finding reliable caregivers requires effort, but it will be worth it!

BE AS FLEXIBLE AS GUMBY

Children change. What works this week to give you and your husband time alone may be obsolete in two months. One couple we know nick-named their children "wedgies" because whenever the parents tried to steal a kiss, the children would wedge between them, grabbing for attention.

You have to grab intimacy with each other, anywhere, anytime. Having young children underfoot requires that you make "Flexible" your middle name. It also helps if you make "Laughter" your first name. When your toddler starts barking like a seal with croup at the moment of orgasm, what else can you do but laugh together? When your son gets up to go to the bathroom but misses the bathroom and goes in your shoe, what can you do but laugh together? When you plan a candlelit dinner just for two and your angel daughters appear saying, "We want candles too," what can you do but smile, promise them candles the next day, and laugh together.

We've discussed the need to make sex a priority. We offered in-home and away-from-home ideas. We've discussed the need to laugh and be flex-ible. But we would be remiss if we failed to bring up one of the most important things you can do to enhance romance: Pray.

PRACTICAL PRAYERS

We know. You'd love to pray. But how can you find time for prayer when you can barely find time to go to the bathroom! Dear tired friend, before you give up, consider the following thoughts about prayer.

1. Thank-you prayers. We are instructed to "Always [give] thanks for all things in the name of our Lord Jesus Christ to God, even the Father" (Ephesians 5:20). "All things" includes the struggle of keeping your sex life alive during the "mommy years." Have you thanked God that you are right where you are, knee-deep in diapers, carpools, and hectic activity? Have you thanked Him that it is possible to grow in your sexual relationship with your husband, even during the diaper days?

2. Breath prayers. The Bible says "pray without ceasing" (1 Thessalonians 5:17). It does not say "cease everything and pray." God wants us to learn how to pray in the midst of our activity. As you change the baby's diaper, stop and thank God for your sexual love that created this precious child. When you play a game with your daughter, pause and ask God to help you be a playful wife in the bedroom. When you set aside a pair of shoes because your son has outgrown them, praise God for helping you outgrow wrong attitudes or behaviors.

These are "breath" prayers, quick moments of exhaling requests to God and inhaling His holy help. In her book *Diapers, Pacifiers, and Other Holy Things,* Lorraine says that as she began to incorporate breath prayers into her day, a strange thing happened. "I began to sing! In the midst of mundane duties, God was allowing me to glimpse His glory. Even as I wiped spit up off the floor or cleaned strained peas off the wall, I rejoiced. I was in the presence of the living God."[5]

3. Scripture prayers. Write verses such as Proverbs 5:18-19, Song of Solomon 5:16 or 5:1b on 3" x 5" cards and tape them in conspicuous locations: by the changing table, in the bathroom, next to the highchair, on the steering wheel of the car. Then pray the verses back to God. "Lord, Your Word says I am to feast on our sexual love, to drink deeply of the physical joy. Show me how to do this even in the midst of exhaustion" (a prayer paraphrase of Song of Solomon 5:1b).

4. Commitment prayers. God wants us to choose not to be anxious about this stage of life, but instead to take the concerns and lift them to Him in prayer with thanksgiving. He promises that when we do this, His peace will be like a garrison of angels to guard our hearts and minds (Philippians 4:6-7). Will you pray?

> *Lord, it seems impossible to be a creative lover to my husband right now. I confess that I've been groaning instead of being thankful. Please forgive me. And Lord, right now I lift my relationship with my husband to You. I give You all my worries about when and how we can grow together sexually. I leave this with You. Fill me with Your peace and show me practically how to be a creative lover now.*

When you pray like this, you send a message to God that you long to become a godly and sensuous lover—even with kids wrapped around your knees!

CHANGE MY HEART, O GOD

1. Ask your husband to read this chapter. Then, schedule a date and have a heart-to-heart talk about your sexual relationship. (It can even be a late dinner at home after the kids are in bed.) Let him know that you desire to make your love life a priority. Together, go over the ideas in this chapter and decide what you can do together to recharge your sexual batteries.

2. Pick one practical suggestion from the chapter and make it a reality this week.

3. Read through the different types of prayers on pages 75-6. Choose two kinds of prayers to practice this week.

⚮

ADJUST YOUR EXPECTATIONS

Weary parents cannot expect to have "Hollywood sex" every time they get together, but with a littler effort, "now" can be better than "then."

Then: We went to the movies, shared buttered popcorn, and held (salty) hands.

Now: We eat microwave popcorn, snuggle under a blanket, and watch a home video we can "pause" in case of a baby emergency.

Then: We kissed for thirty seconds while our sports car idled at a red light.

Now: We exchange neck massages as we drive the family van cross-country to Grandma's.

Then: We went to a concert and played footsie while the orchestra warmed up.

Now: We play *Phantom of the Opera* on our home stereo system and dance with each other and our child.

Then: We gazed lovingly into each other's eyes over a candlelit meal at a French restaurant.

Now: We share a french fry at McDonald's and laugh as we watch our son play in the colored balls.

Then: We were spontaneous, and it was fun.

Now: We plan, and it's beautiful.

Then: Intimacy just happened.

Now: We make intimacy happen.

part two

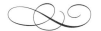

Smoldering Questions

How Can I Get over the Guilt of Past Sexual Sin?

*H*ow great is our need for cleansing—the kind of deep, soaking cleansing that seeps into the crevices of our souls and enables us to proclaim, "I am clean."

We tuck painful memories away in the basement of our hearts where cobwebs and spiders lurk. There they remain, covered by darkness, sealed behind a closed door. Years pass. A foul odor rises from the basement. The stench permeates the house, affecting us and our relationships with our husbands.

Glade spray and potpourri candles won't solve the problem. As difficult as it may be, we must remove what's buried below. God waits, eager to help, but we must be the ones to open the basement door and carry the hidden things out of the darkness and into His light.

I (Lorraine) had just finished outlining this chapter and writing the above paragraphs when the phone rang. I assumed it would be Linda, telling me what time she would be over so we could talk about the sections of the book we were each working on. Instead, it was my longtime friend and walking partner, Christine, who wanted to tell me she'd found a mango-colored blouse at 60 percent off to go with a patchwork vest she'd recently purchased.

"That's terrific, Chris. It will look dynamite with your blazing red hair. Listen, I can't talk now. I'm working fast and furiously on a really important chapter for the book."

"What's it about?"

"How to get over the guilt of past sexual sin."

"I don't think I have a problem with that, but how would I know if I did?"

Christine and I had met at a writer's conference ten years ago and had been kindred spirits ever since. We'd talked about every subject under the sun *except* sex. I knew she'd grown up in a strict Christian home. I knew her husband, Stewart, but I didn't know the specifics of her sexual past. I asked her the first question from my "guilt indicator" questions: Do you believe sex with your husband can be exciting and wonderful, but don't give yourself permission to enjoy it because you feel guilty about things you did in the past?

By the gasp on the other end of the phone, I knew the question rang true. I continued with the other questions:

- Did you feel ashamed walking down the wedding aisle in front of your family wearing white?
- Was your first night together as husband and wife a disappointment because you knew each other too well?
- Do you ever feel angry at yourself or your husband because you compromised your sexual boundaries?
- Do you fantasize about other men while you are making love with your husband and feel remorse that what's going on in your head is more exciting than what's going on in your bed?
- Do you sometimes feel incomplete because you gave part of yourself to other men through sexual intercourse or intimate touching?
- Do you frequently feel sex is overrated, that you could get by fine without it?

Christine was silent. Then a tearful admission, "Lorraine, every one of those statements describes me."

"Girl, grab your walking shoes and get over here now! We've got some praying to do."

As Christine stretched her calf muscles for our "holy hike"—a two-mile, winding mountain path near my home—I explained that cleansing ourselves from past sexual sin is much like taking a shower. First we get rid of the old, like we remove dirty clothes before showering. Next we step under the water and allow God's forgiveness to pour over us and wash our past down the drain. Finally, we put on new, clean garments, which the Bible calls clothing ourselves in the righteousness of Christ (2 Corinthians 5:21, Galatians 3:27).

"Getting rid of the old is usually the hardest part of the cleansing process," I said, "but we all have to go through it. You may think you're alone, Christine, but the majority of Christian women have a sexual history to deal with. Just be honest with God. Admit to Him everything you've done—He already knows it anyway. Tell Him you were wrong and are grieved over your sin. As we walk, I'll be beside you, but don't talk to me, talk to God. Okay?" Christine nodded in agreement. As the gravel crunched beneath our feet, Christine poured out her heart to God.

"Father, first of all, I ask you to forgive me for letting Brad touch me where he shouldn't have. I knew it was wrong, but I liked him so much, and I didn't exactly dislike what he was doing. Still, I'm sorry. I should have stopped him. And please forgive me for letting Craig touch me in a similar way. Why did I do that? I wasn't even attracted to him. Oh yes, I'd almost forgotten Richard in college. He was so charming. I let him get closer than I should have."

As Christine talked, I prayed silently that God would show her all her basement memories, that He would expose every corner. Suddenly there was a pause as she thought of her husband, Stewart. Tears dripped on her Nikes. "God, forgive me for giving in to Stewart before we got married. I wanted to wait. I tried to wait. Why did he push so hard? Why didn't he respect my wishes? It made me so mad. It still makes me mad!"

Choking, Christine sat on the rock I pointed out as a good resting place. Hunched over, hands covering her face, her body shook with sobs. Somewhere in the darkness of her memories, a light switched on and she saw the impact her sexual decisions had made upon her marriage. "Oh, God, what have I done? I've been living as a separate person for all these years. I knew giving in to Stewart was wrong so, even though I gave in physically, I withheld something emotionally and spiritually. I've been married fifteen years, and I've never fully given myself to my own husband! God, is this why our sex life is so crummy?"

Suddenly many of Christine's decisions made sense to her; a separate checking account, her separate identity through her work, why she felt the need to assert herself over her husband rather than yield to him. The anger she felt toward him and toward herself had placed a small gulf between them. "All these years, I've blamed Stewart for the lack of intimacy in our marriage, but now I see I am the one to blame. Forgive me, God," she cried.

I wrapped my arms around my friend and wept with her. A warmth spread over us as the autumn sun broke through the clouds. Light spilled around us, God's grace flowed over us. Christine's bitter tears became cleansing tears as God's forgiveness washed through her.

Several minutes later, she was quiet. "Are you okay?" I asked. She lifted her head, looking like a woeful raccoon with her smudged mascara. She sighed, then smiled a radiant smile, the smile of one who has been touched by the living God.

I picked up a stick. "See this stick? We're going to put it in the ground right here by this rock as a reminder that you have received God's forgiveness. That way, if you ever doubt what happened today—if an old memory creeps into your mind to condemn you—think of this stick and say to that memory, 'I am forgiven.'" I poked the stick in the ground. The bottom snapped off. We laughed at my attempt to make a solid spiritual analogy with such a frail twig. Oh well, short as the stick was, it would serve as a marker, an eternal reminder, of the day God pronounced her clean.

As we headed back home I said, "Christine, God has forgiven you, but you still need to forgive Stewart."

"I know."

"Please, let me know when you do that. And don't wait too long, okay?"

"I won't," she promised, then added thoughtfully. "Lorraine, what happened today was a miracle, wasn't it?"

"Yes, the kind of miracle God wants to do every day for women everywhere."

FORGIVENESS IS FOR YOU TOO

Perhaps as you read about Christine's sexual sins you thought, *She doesn't even begin to know what guilt feels like. I'm too disgusted to even think about what I did. I'd have to walk ten miles to have enough time to name all the men I've been intimate with.* Or maybe you've had a "clean" sexual history and would only have to walk a block, but you know deep in your heart you have a mind filled with wrong attitudes. Wherever you are, whatever you've done, God desires to extend His grace to you.

King David, who committed adultery *and* murder made the following statement:

> Vindicate me, O LORD, for I have led a blameless life; I have trusted in the LORD without wavering. Test me, O LORD, and try me, examine my heart and my mind; for your love is ever before me, and I walk continually in your truth. (Psalm 26:1-3, NIV)

This statement is incredible! How could David say he'd led a blameless life when he'd committed adultery with Bathsheba and then had her husband murdered? David's life demonstrates that no matter how wretched the sin of our past, God is able to declare us blameless.

Would you like to say of yourself, "I am blameless"? You can. Regardless of how terrible the thought or wicked the deed, God can forgive you and wipe the slate clean. How does this happen?

RELEASE THE OLD

The first step in the cleansing process is to release the old. This involves getting rid of every vile memory, every filthy attitude, or immoral act. If you have never given your sexual past to God, never confessed your regret for intimate touching or sexual intercourse outside marriage, we encourage you to do this now.

CAN I BECOME A VIRGIN AGAIN?

A young woman came to us and asked, "I've had sex with four different men. Now that I've gone through the cleansing steps and God has forgiven me for my past, is it possible for me to become a virgin again?"

The word *virgin* means "pure." Even after a woman has yielded her virginity, she can become pure in her sexual thoughts and attitude, in her dress and demeanor, and how she relates to men. The blood of Christ can wash us clean and make our sins white as snow. Such a woman can become a virgin in every way but technically.

You may wonder, *Is it really necessary to go through this "removal" process when I no longer have any physical contact with my former lover?* Yes. Unlike other sins committed "outside the body," sexual sin is a sin committed in the body that makes you "one" with another person physically, emotionally, and spiritually (1 Corinthians 6:15-18). Every person you have ever "given" yourself to has a part of you. Physically, you may have separated from this person, but emotional or spiritual ties may still exist. This explains why you may sometimes feel "incomplete" or grapple with unbidden dreams and longings.

Removing these ties is not complicated. You need only to bring the situation before God, tell Him you are sorry, then ask Him to forgive you and to cut the cords that bind you to the past. It is important to bring each name and sexual act before the Lord so He may cleanse you once and for all. Like Christine, pour out your heart to God. You can do this alone with God or ask a trusted friend to walk through this process with you.

You can make up your own prayer, or you might want to use this prayer that has helped hundreds of women break free from the bondage of their sexual past.[1]

> *Dear Heavenly Father,*
>
> *I know that it was sinful and offensive to You when I committed sexual immorality by (offense) with (name of person). I understand that by this sexual act I joined my spirit together with _____'s spirit. I ask that You forgive me for (offense) and that You will break this spiritual union with _____. Grant me spiritual freedom from _____ and return my spirit to me. I ask that the blood of Jesus would cleanse my spirit as it returns to me. I pray that the door of sensual thought and action toward _____ will be closed forever. Dear God, make me spiritually whole again. This I pray by faith and through the power of Jesus. Amen.*

Cutting ties with former lovers is like removing the big, obvious boxes in your basement. Once you've given these to God, the heavy work is done; the majority of your basement is clean. Now go back and check the corners. Ask God to expose any hidden sin, such as wrong attitudes, immoral thoughts, or unintentional actions that grieved God. Jesus said, "For whatever is hidden is meant to be disclosed, and whatever is concealed is meant to be brought out into the open" (Mark 4:22, NIV).

Like David and Job, pray:

> Teach me what I cannot see. (Job 34:32, NIV)

> Search me, O God, and know my heart; test me and know my anxious thoughts. See if there is any offensive way in me. (Psalm 139:23-24, NIV)

The length of time you spend removing the old depends on how much junk is in your basement. Give God time to work. When you are ready—when your basement is empty and your old piles are in God's hands—move on to the next step: bathing in God's forgiveness.

RECEIVE THE NEW

After you release the old, you must receive the new. Receiving may sound easier than releasing, but for many it's not. Why is receiving difficult? Because we don't deserve what God gives. We commit the sin, but God pays the price. We do what is wrong, then we have to rely on God to make things right. We wait years to tell God we are sorry; He forgives instantly. It doesn't seem fair, and it isn't! But God's love for us is unconditional. Though we fail Him, He always gives, always loves, always reaches out to us. Nothing would grieve God more than for us to reject His love. Nothing would please Him more than for us to embrace His grace. So, undeserving as we are, we must receive what He offers.

A man with leprosy knelt before Jesus, saying, "Lord, if You are willing, You can make me clean" (Matthew 8:2). Jesus touched him and said, "I am willing. Be clean."

Old Testament priests used to immerse themselves in a huge tank of water called "the sea" after they had offered sacrifices (1 Kings 7:23). Imagine their joy as the dirt of the world and the sins of the people were washed away. How gloriously refreshing to splash around in God's forgiveness and experience His cleansing power!

You, too, need to jump into His forgiveness, to immerse yourself. Accept His forgiveness. Allow His grace to wash over you. God has forgiven you. Now, offer yourself this same forgiveness. You must forgive *you!* Feel

His love flow around you and in you. Friend, this is not a trickle of water, but a tremendous outpouring of His mercy!

Part of receiving the new is to adorn yourself with the new clothes God has prepared for you. When you are powdered and perfumed after a shower, you put on clean clothes. God has given you new clothes. "Let me tell you how happy God has made me! For he has clothed me with garments of salvation and draped about me the robe of righteousness" (Isaiah 61:10, TLB).

If you have released the old and received the new, God has forgiven you. You may not look different on the outside (except for smudged mascara and red eyes!), but something on the inside is very different. God desires that the "new" be translated into renewed love and desire for your husband. He desires for you to receive His viewpoint about the gift of sex, in your mind, your heart, and your body. He wants you to be free. Free to be the sensuous woman he created you to be. Free to joyously give and receive sexual love in your marriage.

HOW DOES FORGIVENESS FEEL?

How does it feel to be forgiven? Forgiveness is not a feeling, it's a fact. Either you are forgiven, or you are not. If you have confessed your sin, accepted His forgiveness, and forgiven others as you have been forgiven, you ARE forgiven, regardless of how you feel. But what if you don't see evidence in your life that anything has happened? Does this mean you're not forgiven?

Sometimes God heals instantaneously. For Christine it was as if a veil had been lifted before her eyes. She suddenly saw things differently and had a new desire to view sex the way God views sex. In the days that followed, she

HOW GOD HEALS

God heals different people in different ways. Many people Jesus touched received instant healing (Mark 3:5; 5:29; 5:42; 10:52). Others were healed through a process (Mark 8:22-25, Luke 17:14-15). A commander of the king's army with leprosy had to wash seven times in a river until he was clean (2 Kings 5:14). Whether God has chosen to heal you instantly or through a process, you can be sure of His love and faithfulness to you.

moved forward and forgave her husband for pushing her to have sex before they were married. And she was amazed at what happened—she made love with Stewart more times in the next week than in the previous two months!

It would be nice if all women saw instant changes, but this is not the case. Sometimes God heals through a process. A woman healed in this manner might think, *I'm glad I confessed my sins and accepted God's forgiveness, but I'm not sure any change occurred because I don't feel any different.* In the following days she may even find herself thinking old thoughts from her past, just like before. But if she listens with her heart, she will realize, something IS different. A new thought pops up right next to the old thought that says, *You are forgiven.* By faith, this woman must embrace the new voice and reject the old. As Isaiah 43:18-19 (NIV) says, "Forget the former things; do not dwell on the past. See, I am doing a new thing! Now it springs up; do you not perceive it?" Each time she believes the new and rejects the old, she grows into what God has accomplished in her. It's like the old woman who won ten million dollars in the lottery. She was instantly rich, but it was only as she daily spent what she had received that she was able to say with confidence, "I am a wealthy woman."

However God is healing you, instantly or gradually, trust Him. You have begun the healing process by releasing the old and receiving the new. God's rich mercy has made you a wealthy woman! God longs for you to begin to "spend" your sexual wealth with your husband. As God so beautifully said to the lovers in the Song of Solomon: "Eat, friends; drink and imbibe deeply, O lovers" (5:1).

CHANGE MY HEART, O GOD

1. *Release the old.* Spend an hour alone with God (or with God and a friend) in the cleansing exercise. Meditate on Psalms 51 and 52. For many women, it is helpful to create a physical reminder of the spiritual step they have taken. Christine's stick and rock testify of her cleansing. Later, after she forgave Stewart, she put a stick in a flowerpot and placed it on her bathroom counter. "Whenever I am tempted to hold something against Stewart or to withhold myself sexually, I look at that stick and say, 'I forgave and I have been forgiven. I will not think and act

as I have in the past.'" What physical reminders can you use to verify your forgiveness? Here are some suggestions:

- ☙ Place a *stake* in your flower garden or in a houseplant, and write Psalm 32:5 (NIV) on it, "I acknowledged my sin to you and did not cover up my iniquity . . . and you forgave the guilt of my sin."
- ☙ Place a small pair of *scissors* on the nightstand beside your bed to remind you that God has "cut" your ties to the past.
- ☙ Put together a *puzzle*. Praise God for taking the pieces of your life and making you "whole" again. (Hint: Make sure no pieces of the puzzle are missing; otherwise this could be a frustrating activity!)
- ☙ Clean out your *basement* or a storage closet. Throw out everything that is broken or useless. Then, as you see your orderly area, praise God for cleaning the basement of your soul!

2. *Receive the new.*

- ☙ Buy a new *bathrobe* to remind you that you are robed in the righteousness of Christ. Every time you wrap the soft new robe around you, thank Him that you have received a new mind and heart concerning sex.
- ☙ Write John 15:3 (NIV) on a note card and tape it to your shower: "You are already clean because of the word I have spoken to you."
- ☙ Write a prayer to God thanking Him for His forgiveness. Read the prayer out loud. Your guilt was hidden, your praise and thankfulness must be heard.

I'm Attracted to Another Man! Help?

*Y*ou are attracted to a man who is not your husband. A thousand questions race through your mind. *Is it really so terrible to daydream about another man? Is it a sin to think such things? How can I quit thinking about this person when I seem to have no control over the thoughts that keep popping into my head? Am I the only one feeling this way, or do other Christian women struggle with sexual temptation?*

Shelly came to us with these questions. She and Richard had a good marriage, but the moment she met Dan at church she felt an instant "chemistry." At first she dismissed her intentions toward Dan as harmless flirtation, but before she knew it, she was playing with the idea of having an affair. Read with us from Shelly's journal to see how quickly "innocent" thoughts can turn into dangerous longings.

> **May 4:** Dan is so considerate. Yesterday, as I was walking out of church, he held the door open for me and told me how nice I looked. I can't remember the last time Richard told me I looked pretty.
>
> **May 15:** Richard and I hired Dan to remodel our basement. It will be great having a man around the house who can fix things! I find myself looking forward to his visits.
>
> **May 20:** Dan is having problems with his daughter. I offered some advice, and he was so grateful he gave me a hug. I wanted to hug him back, but I didn't. I'd never do anything to jeopardize my marriage to Richard. Still, it felt good to be appreciated. I often replay that moment in my mind.

June 1: Dan and I are going to lunch today to finalize details on the basement. I feel like a giddy schoolgirl! I've tried on ten different outfits and put on extra perfume. I keep telling myself it's no big deal, it's just business. But while we talk about bathroom fixtures and electrical outlets, I get to look into those laughing, brown eyes. Dan has great eyes.

June 2: Yesterday during lunch, the cheesecake took me by surprise. Offering him a bite of mine seemed harmless, but the moment he tasted it, our eyes locked and ZAP! A million volts of electricity surged between us. Neither of us said anything but we both knew something was different. We had crossed some unseen line and can never go back to just being friends.

June 4: I'm jittery and jumpy. Each time the phone rings, I hope it's Dan. When a car drives by, I look out the window to see if it's he. I'm filled with longing, and it is not for my husband! Help, God! I know this is wrong, but I don't want it to stop.

Shelly came to us in tears. "I can't believe this is happening to me. I'm a Christian. How can I even *think* about being in the arms of another man? Do other women struggle with this?"

We assured Shelly that other women *do* struggle with sexual temptation. We have. So have other Christian teachers and authors we know. So have many of the women who have attended our Bible studies and conferences. In fact, at some point in their lives, most women will face such temptation.

Recently we asked seventeen women in church leadership and two hundred and fifty women at a retreat, "Have you ever found yourself attracted to another man?" What percent of these godly women do you think said yes? Fifty percent? Seventy percent? No. *Ninety percent* admitted to feeling attracted to another man (for all we know, the other ten percent are either fibbing or newly married!).

These statistics shocked Shelly when we shared them with her. "If this is such a common problem, why isn't anyone talking about it?"

People *do* talk about it—*after* the fact. We talk about the prominent pastors, evangelists, and singers who have fallen into sexual sin. We talk about the couple across the street who is getting a divorce because one partner had an affair. We talk about how tragic it is for the children and the faithful spouse. We discuss the impact of infidelity: the house for sale, the ministry in ruins, the church with empty seats. It's as if we've all agreed to some unwritten rule that it's okay to talk about the *consequences* of sexual sin but not its *causes*.

When was the last time you had a heart-to-heart talk with a godly woman about your struggle—or her struggle–with sexual temptation? For Shelly, the answer was "never." So we talked. Shelly wanted to obey God, but she confessed, "Right now thinking about Dan is the greatest joy in my life. How can I give that up?" She had other questions as well:

- Should I continue working with Dan on the basement? (Please! Don't say no.)
- I want to be appreciated and adored by a man. Is that so terrible?
- Have I committed a sin? After all, Dan and I have never even kissed.
- I know going to bed with Dan is wrong, but what harm is there in mentally reliving the hug we shared?
- How do I know when my thoughts and actions have crossed the line from being safe to being sin?
- I believe God led me to talk with you about my struggle. Should I talk with anyone else? Does my husband need to know? Should I tell Dan how I feel?

Shelly needed a crash course in Temptation 101, so we talked with her about some of the things that have helped us when we've faced temptation. In order to have victory over temptation, we must understand what temptation is and how it affects us.

TEMPTATION: THE QUICKSAND OF THE HEART

Temptation is a strong pull that entices us away from godly thinking and into sinful actions. Temptation has a beginning (the initial enticement), an end (death), and several steps in between. As seen in James 1:14-15, each step builds upon the previous step, producing a deadly downward spiral.

Each one is *tempted* when, by his own evil desire, he is dragged away and *enticed.* Then, after desire has conceived, it gives birth to sin; and sin, when it is full-grown, gives birth to *death.* (NIV, emphasis ours)

This verse suggests three distinct steps, or levels, involved in the temptation spiral: *temptation, contemplation,* and *activation.* Shelly's thoughts concerning Dan did not jump from "Dan is nice" (Level 1—*temptation*) to "I'd love to go to bed with him" (Level 3—*activation*). Instead, thoughts built upon thoughts, actions upon actions, until one day Shelly woke up and found herself emotionally in the arms of another man.

Like quicksand, temptation always urges, always pulls, always sucks us deeper into its depths. The moment we step into it, we feel a steady, downward tug on our ankles. Initially, we can free ourselves by resisting the pull and stepping back onto solid ground. But the longer we stay in, the deeper we sink, until we are in over our heads.

Each level of temptation contains different qualities and dangers, as seen in the following soil analysis.

Level	Soil Name	Sink Factor	Sin Factor
1	Temptation	Up to your ankles	No sin
2	Contemplation	Up to your waist	Stuck in sin
3	Activation	Over your head	Death

Let's look at these three steps as they relate to Shelly's situation.

1. Temptation: Temptation comes to us through our thoughts. Shelly thought, *It sure would be nice to have a considerate man around the house who complimented me and could even fix things.* Her thoughts tempted her to admire Dan and his abilities, to focus on her husband's shortcomings, and to feel cheated that she didn't have a considerate husband who was handy with a wrench. Did Shelly sin by thinking these things? No. It's what Shelly did with the thoughts that opened the door to sin. Instead of immediately saying no to dwelling on Dan's attributes and her husband's shortcomings, she said yes. Saying yes caused her to sink to the next level.

2. Contemplation: In contemplation, we sin by giving ourselves permission to dwell on wrong thoughts and rationalize wrong choices. Shelly said yes to trying on ten different outfits and to going to lunch with Dan. She rationalized her decision by telling herself, *This is just a business lunch—no harm in that.* Suddenly she found herself with the emotionally charged piece of cheesecake she wrote about in her journal.

We do not sin because we are unable to avoid it. We sin because we rationalize and lie to ourselves. We sin because we are selfish, wanting what we want when we want it. We sin because our hearts are deceitful and wicked (Jeremiah 17:9). Shelly was sinking in sin; she needed to get out quickly to avoid death.

3. Activation: In this phase, we act upon our thoughts in direct disobedience to God's commandments. We typically think of activation in terms of outward actions, but we can also activate through inward intentions. For example, we may say, "It's okay for me to imagine making love with this person (inward intention), after all, I'd never actually *do* anything" (outward action). But God does not make such distinctions. Both are equally wrong. Jesus said we commit adultery just by looking at another person with lustful thoughts (Matthew 5:28).

Jesus' statement reveals God's heart: Do not—even in your mind—defile yourself by uniting yourself with a man who is not your husband. When you fantasize about another man while you are making love with your husband, you bring that man into your bed just as surely as if he were physically there. We have seen numerous situations in which a husband or wife has a "best friend" of the opposite sex. The relationship between the two involves intimate sharing and the meeting of needs, yet they feel they are not in error because they don't take off their clothes. This constitutes an emotional affair and robs the marriage of the oneness God intended to be between husband and wife.

Just how far can we go in thought and action before we fall into sexual sin? Our human nature always seeks to get away with as much as is legally possible. We give ourselves permission to flirt, vowing never to cross the line into lust. We toy with temptation and indulge in contemplation, assuring ourselves we will pull out before "things get out of hand." But we deceive ourselves. We are never safe. We never know which temptation, which thought or action, will pull us across the line into sin. It can happen with frightening speed. It's like the three-year-old who innocently explains how she came to be eating the cookie from the cookie jar: "I just climbed up on the counter to smell the cookies and my tooth got caught."

Make no mistake: There's no room for fooling around. If you play with fire, you *will* get burned—and so will those closest to you. Consider the seriousness of your thoughts and actions and make a choice to say no to the temptation facing you. A good place to begin is with prayer. Won't you pray 1 Corinthians 10:13?

> No temptation has overtaken you but such as is common to man. *Thank You, Jesus, that I am not the only person who has ever suffered this way, that You also know what it feels like to be tempted.*
>
> And God is faithful, who will not allow you to be tempted beyond what you are able. *Lord, You know how weak I am. Thank You for Your promise never to give me more than I can handle.*
>
> . . . but with the temptation will provide the way of escape. *God, you've made a way of escape. What is it? Please show me.*

TEMPTATION CHASERS

Here are some techniques that have worked for women in battling temptation:

- "When wrong thoughts of my former boyfriend popped into my head, I willfully replaced those thoughts with mental images of him enjoying an evening with his wife and kids."
- "I did a lot of role playing. I mentally carried out the affair to its logical conclusion. When I pictured the disgust in my children's eyes when they learned what Mom was doing, when I visualized the fallen countenances of those I loved, I knew I had to stop before it was too late. I also imagined what headline might be written in the future about me. 'Mother of Three Abandons Children and Husband for Younger Man.' This was not how I wanted my life to read."
- "My kids brought me back to earth. I wanted Jim, but I wanted the respect of my kids more. I knew both weren't possible."

ESCAPE ROUTES

God provides many ways of escaping sexual temptation. We will look at six. Your own escape may be one of these or it may be one uniquely designed by God just for you. The way of escape is not the important thing; what matters is that *you are always looking for an escape and quickly take it before it passes you by.*

1. Flee. "Flee immorality" (1 Corinthians 6:18). Get out. Now. This verse is a command, not a suggestion. Flee temptation and leave no forwarding address. Proverbs 5:8 warns, "Keep your way far from [him], and do not go near the door of [his] house."

Fleeing often means taking drastic measures. For one woman, it meant exchanging her gallant thirty-five-year-old physician for a portly practitioner. For another it meant giving up a job she loved. Still another told us it meant losing the friendship of the man she felt attracted to. For Shelly it meant turning over the basement project to Richard, and leaving the house whenever Dan had an appointment to be there.

2. Tell a friend. "Confess your sins to one another . . . that you may be healed" (James 5:16). As long as something remains hidden, it has power, but when we bring our secret out into the open, its power is broken. Confessing your desires to a trustworthy friend is like removing the teeth from an angry dog. Temptation may still hound you, but the bite is gone.

After Shelly shared her secret with us, an enormous weight lifted from her shoulders. We prayed with her and agreed to call her once a week for the next several months. "Your accountability and encouragement made it easier to do what was right," she said.

Is there someone you feel comfortable with, someone you can trust who will give you godly wisdom? Ask this person to hold you accountable. Tell her your struggles. You may also want to talk to your church counselor or Bible study leader. But NEVER, NEVER, NEVER talk to "him." Confiding in "him" is like throwing gasoline on a fire.

3. Set boundaries. Decide ahead of time what you will and won't do. Many factors influence boundaries; cultural settings, age, personality type, and personal convictions. While boundaries will vary from person to person, the boundaries you set should reinforce biblical commands such as

- Avoid the appearance of evil. (1 Thessalonians 5:22)
- Do not cause others to stumble by your actions. (2 Corinthians 6:3)
- Be self-controlled and pure. (Titus 2:5)
- Do not let even a hint of sexual immorality characterize your behavior; no obscenity, foolish talk, or coarse joking. (Ephesians 5:3-4)

Here are some boundaries women have shared with us:

"If I am having lunch or dinner with a man other than my husband, I always try to have another woman present. Of course, my father and eighty-nine-year-old uncle are excluded from this rule!"

"I avoid watching movies or reading books that promote immoral sexual relationships so I am less tempted to look at other men in a way that is wrong."

"I dress to please God. Before I leave my house I ask myself, 'Would God approve of how I look?'"

"When an impure thought about another man crosses my mind, I *immediately* cast it out and ask God's forgiveness."

"I no longer enter into sexual jokes and innuendoes. I nip such talk in the bud by walking away or changing the subject."

A stay-at-home mother we know has set this boundary for herself:

"I will not put myself in a position where I see a man other than my husband for five consecutive days." (When you are around toddlers twenty-four hours a day, even men with body odor and no teeth can appear inviting!)

A well-known speaker adds this boundary:

"I will not hug other men. If I sense a man wants to hug me, I immediately extend my hand for a handshake." (This tactic is officially known as 'hug diversion.')

Jean, a sales representative whose work requires she travel with men, shares these boundaries:

> "On business trips, I carry two pictures of my husband with me, one for my purse, the other for the nightstand in the hotel room. Having my husband's face before me wards off wrong thoughts about other men. I inform my male associates I am unavailable for dinner meetings unless it is with a group of people and the purpose of the gathering is business."

Certain "seasons" of life require more stringent boundaries than others. A woman experiencing a "winter" in her marriage, a time when her relationship with her husband feels cold and dead, needs to take extra precautions because of her vulnerability. A woman entering the "autumn" of her life (forty or older) often seeks affirmation from men that even though she is "over the hill" she is still desirable. Under such circumstances, tighter boundaries may be required.

An occasion to bump into an "old flame" is another reason to buttress the boundaries. We know a woman who went to her fiftieth high-school reunion and danced with her first love. She said, "After the dance, I had to literally run away because the old feelings were still there." This from a sixty-eight-year-old happily married woman!

We cannot be too careful when it comes to dealing with someone for whom we've felt an attraction. Once you've experienced an emotional current with another man, the potential for electricity is always there. Boundaries will vary depending upon individual personality and circumstance, but we all need boundaries, not just for the moment of temptation but for a lifetime.

4. Gouge out your eye. "What? Linda, Lorraine, you've got to be joking. Are you telling me to gouge out my eye just because I like looking at other men?" That depends. How long are you looking, and what is going on in your mind while you look? Listen to Jesus' warning.

> If your right eye causes you to sin, gouge it out and throw it away. It is better for you to lose one part of your body than for your whole body to be thrown into hell. And if your right hand causes you to sin, cut it

off and throw it away. It is better for you to lose one part of your body than for your whole body to go into hell. (Matthew 5:29-30, NIV)

Why does Jesus make these radical statements? First, He wants to make it clear that we are to cut off whatever causes us to sin. *Cut off* your relationship with this man. *Chop off* every thought and mental image of him the instant it enters your mind. Second, Jesus wants to emphasize that sexual sin leads to death. Physical death, spiritual death, the death of your marriage. When you desire another man, you kill marital trust and risk the judgment of God.

5. Practice spiritual disciplines. Satan is called "the tempter." He will tempt you, just as he tempted Jesus. The best way to defeat the tempter is through Scripture memorization, prayer, and fasting.

For forty days Jesus submitted himself to Satan's grueling temptations (Matthew 4:1-11). He was tempted in *all* things—this means in all probability He was sexually tempted by a woman—yet He did not sin (Hebrews 4:15). Amazing. How did He do it?

Each time Jesus was tempted He wielded His sword, God's Word. "The word of God is living and active and sharper than any *two-edged sword*" (Hebrews 4:12, emphasis ours). Jesus slashed Satan's temptations to bits by declaring: "It is written . . ." After Jesus spoke God's Word, "the devil left Him" (Matthew 4:11).

In addition to speaking God's Word, Jesus employed two other spiritual disciplines during His temptation: prayer and fasting. In his excellent book *The Power of Prayer and Fasting*, Ronnie Floyd says that prayer and fasting are gateways to God's supernatural intervention.[1] When practiced as God intended, prayer and fasting have the ability to break bondages that cannot be broken through any other means. When the disciples complained they could not cast out a certain demon, Jesus said, "This kind can come out *only* by prayer [and fasting]" (Mark 9:29, NIV, emphasis ours).

Is there power in prayer and fasting? Absolutely! We were told of a woman on an airplane who noticed the man sitting next to her refused his "delightful airplane meal."

"Aren't you hungry?" she asked the man.

"No, I'm fasting," he replied.

"Oh, are you a Christian?" she inquired.

"No, I'm a Satanist. We Satanists are committed to fast and pray that the marriages of Christian leaders will fail."

Consider the number of Christian leaders who have succumbed to sexual temptation, and ask yourself whether their fasting and prayers have been successful. Friend, do not be deceived. Satan—and those who follow him—would love nothing more than to see Christian marriages destroyed. One of Satan's most effective weapons of destruction is sexual temptation.

James 4:7 says, "Resist the devil and he will flee from you." The next time you find yourself desiring another man, boldly rebuke the enemy by praying out loud, "Satan, in the name of Jesus Christ, I command you to flee." Though the devil may return to tempt you again, as he did with Jesus, be assured if you continue to rebuke him, he will depart (Matthew 4:11).

6. Redirect your passion. Shelly had a severe case of misplaced passion. We encouraged her to take the feelings she had for Dan and transfer them back to her husband. (Refer to chapter 10 for more information on how to remain faithful in a faithless world.) Several things helped her in this process. First, she took a trip down memory lane by reviewing her wedding photos and some old love letters from Richard. Then she compiled a list of reasons why she married Richard and made a commitment to focus on his strengths rather than his shortcomings. She spent a great deal of time in prayer asking God to give her new eyes with which to see her husband. Her marriage to Richard is still not perfect, but it is improving all the time.

WHEN NOTHING WORKS

What happens when nothing seems to terminate the temptation?

One friend shared, "I've been struggling with an emotional affair for years. I've tried self-discipline, prayer, memorizing Scripture, talking to my pastor—you name it, I tried it. But any relief I experienced was only temporary. Despite my best efforts, the longings returned. I'm so weary. I don't know how much longer I can continue to fight this fight."

Author Charles Mylander struggled with sexual temptation for many years. In his book *Running the Red Lights: Putting the Brakes on Sexual Temptation,* he writes, "What did it take to win on the battleground of my life? It took all the grace of God I could possibly grab hold of. It took an ever-deepening dependence on Christ and His power. Then it took all the self-discipline I could somehow muster. On top of all of this it took tireless diligence and unending determination day after day after day."[2]

Another battle-weary sufferer, Jenny, adds. "One day I fell to the floor on my face and cried out to Jesus, 'Lord, I know you faced sexual temptation because the Bible says you were tempted in *every* way. But you didn't sin. You didn't give in to the temptation. I wish I could say the same, but I can't. Help! I need a fresh work of Your Spirit. Please, Lord Jesus, be my victor.'"

If you have tried everything and are still failing, let Jesus be your victor. Don't try to accomplish in your flesh what can only be accomplished by God's Spirit. "'Not by might nor by power, but by my Spirit,' says the LORD Almighty" (Zechariah 4:6, NIV).

A FINAL WARNING

Jesus' warning in Matthew 26:41 is worthy of consideration: "Watch and pray so that you will not fall into temptation" (NIV). We must prayerfully guard our hearts when it comes to sexual temptation because, like a pendulum, our attitude often swings from one extreme to the other. In the presence of severe temptation, inadequacy assails us, and we feel certain we, too, will fall. In the absence of temptation, we pridefully believe our "strong marriage" or "noble character" will prevent us from ever committing sexual sin. Both attitudes are wrong. Both invite disaster.

If we are ever to curtail the widespread devastation caused by sexual sin, we must bring the pendulum back to the middle, to the lowest point of the swing, and humble ourselves before God. In brokenness, we must acknowledge the deceitfulness of our hearts, place *no* confidence in the flesh and *all* confidence in God who is able to keep us from falling.

CHANGE MY HEART, O GOD

1. Read Genesis 3:1-8. Consider Eve's temptation in light of the progressive steps outlined in this chapter. First, Satan encouraged Eve to look at the fruit God had forbidden, telling her that eating it would make her as wise as God (Temptation). Eve pondered the thought, then picked the fruit and rationalized why she should say yes to eating it (Contemplation). Finally, in direct disobedience to God, she ate (Activation).

2. The root of Eve's temptation was that she believed God was denying her something she deserved. She doubted God's goodness. Could this be the root of Shelly's problem? Could this be the root of all temptation?

3. The results of Eve's sin were guilt and shame (Genesis 3:7) and broken fellowship with God (Genesis 3:8). Aren't these *always* the consequences of yielding to temptation? Are you willing to risk these consequences for momentary pleasure?

How Can I Remain Faithful
in a Faithless World?

*E*mma flipped through the Saturday paper, pausing at the anniversary announcements. A familiar couple caught her eye. She knew the Brewers from church. Fifty years of marriage. Amazing. Pictures of other silver-haired seniors beamed at her, all celebrating golden anniversaries. One thing was certain, she'd never see Gretchen's picture on the "Fifty Year" page. Her high-school friend had phoned yesterday, informing her that her divorce was final. After eighteen years of marriage, she was leaving her husband for a man that "understood her."

Emma knew others who'd never make the page. Her neighbor. Her daughter's math teacher. Even her mother. All were divorced because one partner in the marriage had been unfaithful.

Would her picture ever appear on the "Fifty Year" page? Her marriage to Michael had had its ups and downs. She'd never cheated on him, although on several occasions she'd been tempted. Next year they would celebrate their twenty-fifth anniversary. Plans were already underway for a cruise to Alaska. The silver celebration was "in the bag." But the golden? She'd known several couples—*Christian* couples she would have described as Mr. and Mrs. Perfect—who had divorced. If those couples hadn't made it, what chance did she and Michael have?

She put down the paper, deep in thought. *With all the pressures and temptations pulling at my marriage, how can I faithfully love and cherish this one man for fifty years? Or longer?*

⁓⦇⦈⁓

On our wedding day, we (Linda and Lorraine) vowed in the presence of God, family, and friends to be faithful to our husbands until "death do us part." We all know couples who made similar vows and ended up divorced. Fifty years ago, divorce was rare. Today more than one million marriages in the United States are dissolved each year because of divorce. A Gallup Poll shows that only 17 percent of marriages actually end because of adultery. A whopping 47 percent end because of "incompatibility."[1] What is going on? Why are couples treating their marriage covenants so lightly? Why are they rejecting the vows they once uttered with such passionate conviction?

We are convinced the number one reason for the escalating divorce rate among Christian couples is that they are embracing the world's mind-set, rather than God's mind-set, regarding their marriage vows. Let's take a closer look at what this means.

THE WORLD'S MIND-SET

We live in a world that values convenience over permanence. Societal attitudes are vastly different today than in the days of the 1950s television show *I Love Lucy.* We have temporary licenses, temporary visas, and temporary addresses. We expect instant cash, fast food, quick fixes, and instant great sex. We purchase disposable goods and refundable merchandise. We walk up, drive through, and exit through the door on the left. We abhor suffering, not only for the pain it brings, but for the inconvenience. The only thing worse than having an ailment we can't numb is standing in line for *five whole minutes* to fill a prescription!

We live in a world that devalues promises. "No new taxes," politicians pledge. "Satisfaction Guaranteed!" advertisements announce. Marketing copy promises products will be "long-lasting and durable." We've been disappointed so many times in so many ways by broken promises that we no longer expect promises to be honored. As a result, we are skeptical and distrustful of promises made to us and disloyal to the promises we make to others.

We live in a world that views happiness as a "right." People emerged from the Great Depression with an attitude of long-suffering and forbearance.

They'd experienced the worst of times, and while they yearned for happiness, they did not see happiness as something owed to them. Today the fast-track, upwardly mobile society in which we live has produced a breed of impatient people demanding immediate gratification. We've somehow translated our constitutional right to pursue happiness as the right to possess happiness. Advertising slogans daily reinforce this notion. "You deserve a break today." "If it feels good, do it." "Pamper yourself . . . you are worth it."

In a society that devalues permanence, distrusts promises, and demands happiness, the prevailing mind-set toward *things* is if it's old, throw it away. If it's not convenient, forget it. If it's promised, don't expect it. If it makes you happy, use it. Unfortunately, this thinking has infected our attitude toward *relationships*. A husband throws away his marriage because it has grown old. A wife says, "Forget it," because loving her husband has become inconvenient. We break promises and justify divorce and extramarital affairs with thoughts such as, *I have a right to be happy. I have a right to be understood and to have my needs met.*

Where does such thinking lead? One wife summarizes it well in a letter to Ann Landers.

> Dear Ann Landers: Sometimes you feel lonely and unloved in a marriage—even after twenty-three years. You feel as if there's got to be more to life, so you set out to find someone who can make you blissfully happy. You believe you have found that someone and decide he is exactly what you want. So you pack up and say good-bye to your twenty-three-year marriage and all the friends you made when you were part of a couple. You give your children the option of coming with you or staying with their father.
>
> You live the glorious life for a few years, and then a light bulb goes on in your empty head. You realize that you have exactly the life you had before—the only difference is that you've lost your friends, your children's respect and the best friend you loved and shared everything with for twenty-three years. And you miss him.
>
> You realize that love doesn't just happen, it must be nurtured through the years. You cannot undo what has been done, so you settle for a lonely and loveless life with emptiness in your heart.

Ann, please print my letter so others won't give up something that is truly precious—and let them know that they won't know how precious it is until they have thrown it away.

—Heavy-hearted in Philly[2]

Is there anything we can do to keep from ending up like this wife? Yes. We can reject the world's mind-set of disposable relationships, empty promises, and self-centered thinking and embrace God's mind-set of permanence, faithfulness, and Christ-centered living.

GOD'S MIND-SET

To God, forever does not mean "for as long as the marriage works." Forever means for the rest of our lives. God sees our vows as life-binding, permanent.

> This is what the LORD commands: When a man makes a vow to the LORD or takes an oath to obligate himself by a pledge, he must not break his word but *must do everything* he said. (Numbers 30:1-2, NIV, emphasis ours)

Jesus commands, "Do not break your oath, but keep the oaths you have made to the Lord. . . . let your 'Yes' be 'Yes' and your 'No,' 'No,'" (Matthew 5:33,37, NIV). God says, "I hate divorce." He warns those who forsake their vows to expect serious consequences (Malachi 2:13-16).

Perhaps at this point you'd like to stop reading. You don't want to hear how seriously God takes your vows because you'd like to get out of them. Your marriage is an empty shell, a farce. There's no sense in continuing on because nothing will ever change. (Oops! There's that world mind-set again. "I want happiness, and I want it NOW!")

Friend, a marriage where the husband and wife love each other sacrificially does not happen overnight. Growing in oneness is a process. Growing in sexual intimacy is a process. Learning how to glorify God and serve each other in your marriage is not something that comes about with the snap of our fingers. Many couples vow, "For better, for worse; for richer, for poorer; in sickness and in health," but when "worse," "poorer," and "sickness" descend, they check out. Yet these trials could have been the very thing God intended to bring about the rich relationship for which they longed.

Marriages are never stagnant; they are always going somewhere. If a marriage is neglected, it will follow the principle of deterioration, which says all things (our bodies, our homes, and yes, our marriages) tend toward decay. But if a marriage is daily nurtured and tended, it will flourish. Are you willing to work on your marriage? Are you determined to fulfill your marriage vows even when everything inside you screams you don't want to?

Persevere, God urges. In perseverance, the hope of your first love can be restored. God commended the Ephesians for their perseverance, but corrects them for straying from their first love (Christ). The following passage points out three Rs that will help them return to their first love: *remember, repent,* and *return.*

> You have perseverance and have endured for My name's sake, and have not grown weary. But I have this against you, that you have left your first love. *Remember* therefore from where you have fallen, and *repent* and [*return* and] do the deeds you did at first. (Revelation 2:3-5, emphasis ours)

This scripture also applies to our marriages. Because we are Christians, some of us have persevered. (We're still married after all these years.) God commends this. But like the Ephesians, we have lost our first love and settled for mediocrity. The passion of our early longings has been replaced with lukewarm affection. How do we return to the fervor of first love? We remember, repent, and return.

REMEMBER FROM WHERE YOU HAVE FALLEN

To keep the fires of first love burning, we must go back to the place where love began, back to the moment we said "I do." The Pintuses have been married for nineteen years, the Dillows for thirty-five. So for us, remembering means brushing away a few mental cobwebs. Still . . .

Lorraine Remembers

The church was packed. I stood at the doorway of the sanctuary feeling like a princess in my flowing white gown. A sheer veil cascaded down my back like a waterfall and spilled into a pool behind me. The "Wedding March" began. Everyone stood. My heart swelled with emotion as I surveyed the familiar faces. An old high-school friend. A new friend from work. College sorority sisters. The family I'd known forever and the family I'd soon come to know. It was as if past, present, and future had merged together to witness this glorious moment, the moment in which I would become Mrs. Peter Pintus.

Peter waited eagerly at the end of the aisle. We drank each other in with our eyes. Deep rivers of love flowed between us. Peter filled empty places in my soul. He made me feel whole. In some ways, I felt as if I'd known him all my life. (Was it possible we'd known each other less than a year?)

I uttered my vows with such gusto that snickers rippled across the sea of people behind us. I didn't care. I wanted them to hear! I wanted the whole world to know how much I loved this man! I could imagine no greater joy than to spend the rest of my life with him.

Linda Remembers

Jody grinned like a Cheshire cat as I walked toward him. It was a grin that said, "Wow, she's mine!" I slipped my arm through his. I felt so loved, so desired.

I'd written and memorized my vows. Each word had been carefully chosen to reveal my passion and commitment. As I promised in front of all those witnesses to be faithful to God and to Jody, a sense of reverence crept over me. It was a holy moment. I'd known other couples whose marriages had grown stale, but ours never would! I was determined that our love would always be vibrant and alive. We would never allow our marriage to sink into mediocrity. Passion oozed from our pores, and I vowed it would never be otherwise.

At the reception, Jody pressed his body close to mine. He whispered, "When can we get out of here and be alone?" The sexual energy between us was enough to light a city! As far as I was concerned, forever in his arms wouldn't be time enough.

Now It's Your Turn

Think back to your wedding day. Where did you get married? What time of year was it? What were you wearing? Were you nervous? Excited? What was your groom wearing? What was he feeling? What hopes and dreams did the two of you share?

Who was present to witness your marriage? What did you feel when you spoke your vows? What emotions filled your heart when your groom slipped the ring on your finger and kissed you in front of all those people? How did it feel to be introduced as husband and wife?

If you are having trouble remembering, we encourage you to find your wedding photos and study each picture. If you have a video or audiotape of your wedding, review it. As you look and listen, ask God to open the eyes and ears of your heart to help you remember the passion you shared. Ask the Lord to take you back to the moment you looked in your groom's eyes and spoke your vows. Try to recall the determination you felt to love this man, to make him happy, and to be the wife he needed. Soak in these memories awhile. Then, when remembering is complete, consider R number two: repent.

Repent from Your Present Attitude and Practices

Repent means to do an about-face, to turn from the current direction. If we don't take the time to remember "from where we have fallen," we are tempted to believe that we have nothing from which to repent. We think, *I don't need to repent. I haven't filed for divorce. I've never been sexually unfaithful. I have fulfilled my vows to my husband and God.* But is this true?

Faithfulness to our vows is more than the *absence* of an affair or the *absence* of a divorce document. Faithfulness is the *presence* of love, devotion, honor, loyalty, and encouragement. Faithfulness is positive and dynamic; it means we actively seek the welfare of our spouse. To say "I've been faithful" because I've never committed adultery is to miss entirely God's meaning of faithfulness.

Lewis Smedes, professor of theology at Fuller Theological Seminary writes, "A man or woman can be just too busy, too tired, too timid, too prudent, or too hemmed in with fear to be seriously tempted by an adulterous affair. But this same person can be a bore at home, callous to the delicate needs of his partner. He or she may be too prudish to be an adventuresome lover, but too cowardly to be in honest communication and too busy to put himself out for anything other than a routine ritual of personal commitment."[3]

You may not cheat on your husband with another man, but do you cheat on him by withholding yourself sexually and emotionally? You may not rob your spouse by engaging in an adulterous affair, but do you rob him by allowing your marriage and your sexual relationship to sink into mediocrity and routine?

When faithfulness is defined in these terms, we both confess: We have failed to be faithful.

Lorraine Repents

Sometimes when Peter wants to make love, I roll my eyes and silently moan, *Not again!* I've always got at least ten reasons why this isn't a good time, but truthfully, my reasons are simply another way of saying, "What I want is more important than what you want." This attitude is wrong. I must ask God (and my husband) to forgive me and make the choice to be thankful that I'm married to a man who desires me and delights in making love to me.

Linda Repents

I vowed to make my husband my first priority after God, but sometimes I get so wrapped up in my own projects and pressures, that I fail to stop and look at life through Jody's eyes. It requires time and emotional effort to understand his perspective. There are days I just don't want to go that extra mile. When this happens, I ask God to help me be sensitive to what Jody is thinking and feeling.

We All Fall Short

On our honeymoons, all of us were eager to see life through our spouse's eyes, eager to love him. We hopped out of bed (or lingered in bed depending on the situation), anxious to show our devotion. The distance between "how can I please you" and "don't bother me with sex" is a pretty steep drop.

We all fall short of the glory of God (Romans 3:23). We all fall short of the lofty love we pledged on our wedding day. We all need to repent, to do an about-face in thought and deed.

Sheila needed to repent for mentally "giving up" on her husband. Debbie needed to repent for allowing her sexual relationship to become stale. Molly needed to repent for having an affair. What about you? Is there any area of thinking or acting in which God wants you to do an about-face? This is a prayer we've prayed many times. Perhaps you'd like to pray it now.

> *God, forgive me for slacking off, for not loving my husband with the fervor which I vowed the day we married. Please restore in me the passion of first love and give me the strength to demonstrate that love to my husband.*

RETURN AND DO THE DEEDS YOU DID AT FIRST

Doing the deeds we did at first restores "first love." Remember the old tricks, author and psychologist Dr. James Dobson suggests. "How about breakfast in bed? A kiss in the rain? Or rereading those old love letters together? A night in a nearby hotel? Roasting marshmallows by an open fire? A phone call in the middle of the day? A long-stemmed red rose and a love note?"[4]

Are you willing to put forth effort to have the kind of marriage you dream of? If so, we challenge you to do something concrete to show your love for your husband every day for the next month. One day you might scribble in lipstick on the bathroom mirror, "I love you." Another day, give your husband a five-minute neck massage after dinner. Do one small thing each day, or try something bigger, like some of the practical suggestions offered in chapters 15 and 19. A month is a short time to do these things, and it can make a tremendous difference in your relationship.

If the thought of doing something each day overwhelms you, modify the challenge and plan a "weekly special." We also recommend a "yearly checkup," a "state of the marriage union" event. Here are some things we do each year.

Lorraine and Peter's Anniversary Getaway

Our anniversary is a top priority. Most of our married life, making ends meet has been a fiscal adventure. We cut coupons, shop at garage sales, and have "at home" haircuts, but we never scrimp when it comes to celebrating our anniversary. Our anniversary getaway is nearly always the highlight of our year, due in part to the simple rules we've followed.

- Go away for a minimum of two nights.
- Experience something new together.
- Set aside time for intimacy.

On our seventh anniversary, we splurged on our dream vacation and walked hand in hand on the beaches of Hawaii. (We conceived our first child on this excursion.) Our tenth anniversary found us in a secluded seaside bed-and-breakfast. Anniversary fourteen was spent hiking ten miles of mountain trail rated "most beautiful" by a Colorado tourist group. Anniversaries are an adventure because we always see or do something neither of us has done before. These new memories are like cement poured over the original foundation of our marriage, keeping us on sure footing.

We try to be creative in the sexual area as well. We often abstain from sex the week before our getaway to heighten the anticipation of being together. We always give each other one small gift to enhance romance. Last year Peter gave me a CD of romantic piano music; I gave him purple silk boxer shorts. We always take time to talk, whether it's over dinner, on a hike, or nestled in each other's arms in front of a fire. We reminisce about our favorite anniversary, share goals and dreams, and talk about where we'd like to go next year to celebrate our love. We always conclude our getaway by reaffirming each other's incredible insight in selecting a mate.

Linda's Marriage Statement

At least once a year, I review my personal marriage statement. My marriage statement is an amplification of the vows I made on my wedding day. I go over them each year around our anniversary. Currently it reads as follows (I revise it occasionally as my "resolves" keep growing!):

I RESOLVE to keep Jody my second priority (after God).

I RESOLVE not to settle for mediocrity in my marriage.

I RESOLVE to look at life through my spouse's eyes.

I RESOLVE to grow as a sensuous lover.

I RESOLVE to give rather than to receive.

I RESOLVE to be faithful to my marriage vows, not only in word, but in intent.

THE FOURTH R

Enjoying a great marriage doesn't just happen. Both of us—along with our spouses—have to work at it. We have to regularly *remember, repent,* and *return.* (Especially repent!) But as we've followed these three Rs, God has blessed us with another R, one that makes the investment of effort worthwhile.

The fourth R is Reward. Following God's admonition to *remember, repent,* and *return,* God promises that those who are faithful will receive a *reward,* "the right to eat from the tree of life" (Revelation 2:7, NIV). God says, "In my faithfulness I will reward them," (Isaiah 61:8, NIV). As we are faithful to fulfill our vows, God is faithful to reward us. He blesses us with earthly rewards—stronger character and a richer marriage—but He also promises heavenly rewards (Matthew 16:27, Ephesians 6:8). What greater joy could we desire than to come to the end of our lives and hear the Lord say, "Well done, good and faithful servant. Come and receive your reward" (see Matthew 25:21,23, NIV).

But being faithful is difficult. At times, you will find yourself thinking, *Why do I always have to be the one to make our marriage better? Why do I always have to be the giving and forgiving one? This man is impossible to live with. How can I faithfully love and cherish him and give him my best when he seems bent on showing me his worst?*

From a human standpoint, it is impossible to remain faithful. "With men this is impossible, but with God all things are possible" (Matthew 19:26).

God is able to keep you faithful. God is loyal in His love and devotion to you—loyal to the point of dying for you. He desires to pour His divine love, His divine nature, in you and through you. As you seek Him and yield to Him, He will work in you so you can love your husband.

Faithfulness begins with God. His name is Faithful. When He returns for His bride, the church, He will come riding on a white horse, and His name "is called Faithful and True" (Revelation 19:11). When you feel you can no longer be faithful, He can accomplish faithfulness in you. "Faithful is He who calls you, and He also will bring it to pass" (1 Thessalonians 5:24).

A Song of Faithfulness

Let's return to our original question. Is it possible to remain faithful in a faithless world? Yes. If you trust God and allow Him to work His purposes in your life, if you *remember, repent, return,* then you'll be *rewarded* with an attitude like Aunt Louise's. When asked on her fiftieth wedding anniversary if she ever got bored being with the same man, Aunt Louise smiled and said, "My George is like a piano. On a piano you can play Beethoven's Fifth or 'Happy Birthday.' You can play blues or gospel, ballads or ragtime. You can play a melody that comforts or one that makes you laugh. Bored? No. For me and George, new songs are always in the makin'."

Change My Heart, O God

1. *Remember.* Spend time reviewing your wedding album or watching your wedding video. Then initiate an act of love toward your spouse that you did when you were dating.

2. *Repent.* In what ways have you fallen short of God's intent of faithfulness in your marriage? Pray and ask God to forgive you. Write your husband a note asking forgiveness for not making him your first priority. Tell him you love him and want to honor him as long as you both shall live.

3. *Return.* Write your own marriage statement. You can model it after Linda's or center it around a Bible verse or your original vows. Put it in a picture frame and display it where you can see it.

IF HE'S BEEN UNFAITHFUL . . .

What should you do if your husband has committed the ultimate act of unfaithfulness by sleeping with another woman?

Share. Many women are silent about the affair because they are ashamed and embarrassed, or because they don't want to harm their husband's reputation. But if your husband is having an affair, it is crucial that you have a few *carefully selected* confidants—a trusted friend, pastor, professional counselor, or godly family member—who can ease your emotional burden and help you respond rightly. Your husband needs to be confronted about his sin (Matthew 18:15-17, 1 Corinthians 5:1-2, Galatians 6:1, James 5:19-20). Positive input from family members and the Christian community can strengthen you and influence your husband toward responsible actions. As one "affair survivor" shared, "The best thing I ever did was tell my friend, who prayed with me through that awful year, and my pastor, who talked with my husband and helped him in his decision to end the affair."

Read. First and foremost, spend time in God's Word. "Scripture was my life preserver when I felt like I was drowning," Connie offers. Ponder the book of Hosea, an allegory of how God suffered because of the adulteries of Israel. Grab hold of verses like Jeremiah 29:11 (NIV), "'For I know the plans I have for you,' declares the LORD, 'plans to prosper you and not to harm you, plans to give you hope and a future.'" Bask in the encouragement of Psalms: "God is our refuge and strength, a very present help in trouble" (46:1). In addition to Bible reading, we recommend the excellent books *Love Must be Tough* by Dr. James Dobson (Word Publishing, 1983) and *The Myth of the Greener Grass* by J. Allan Petersen (Tyndale House Publishers, 1996).

Pray. Powerful emotions threaten to undo you: anger, humiliation, fear, and resentment. Your knee-jerk reaction will probably be to lash out. Instead, bend your knee in prayer and seek God's wisdom. He will soothe your emotions and help you respond properly.

Draw the line. "Every wife confronting adultery should insist that her husband sever all connections with the other person and concentrate on enhancing their own marriage satisfaction."[5] Boundaries are critical. One wife told her husband, "If you see her again, the kids and I will leave you." Another said, "No sex until you can give me medical proof that you are free of sexual disease." These are legitimate boundaries; however, your boundaries may be different. As you pray, read, and talk with your trusted confidants, seek wisdom about what boundaries are right for you.

Yield. A wife emerges on the other side of an affair either softened or hardened. If she gives in to her anger and rage, bitterness will harden her. If she yields to God and allows Him to teach and instruct her, wisdom will soften her, and she will become more Christlike. Which will you choose?

No marriage is beyond God's healing touch. Though the pain of adultery can feel like death, God's resurrection power is able to bring life from death. Focus on the Family founder Dr. James Dobson says the tragedy of an affair, "*if properly managed,* can be the vehicle for transforming an unstable relationship into a vibrant, healthy marriage."[6]

eleven

What Do I Do When HE Has a Headache?

*E*rica moaned, "I was sooo tired last night, but as usual, Trevor was ready for fun and games!"

Karen nodded empathetically. "Believe me, I sympathize. When Joel looked at me with that gleam in his eye, I felt like throwing a bucket of cold water on him."

Katie laughed along with her two friends, but inside she was dying. There was no way she could tell two women whose husbands panted at the sight of them that Jason was never ready for fun and games. He never even wanted her. Katie turned her head to hide the tears. *Oh God,* she silently cried, *what is the matter with me? Why doesn't my husband want to make love with me?*

Is this a common problem? More so than you might think.

THE PROBLEM NO ONE TALKS ABOUT

As I (Linda) walked into the main room of the retreat center, my eye was immediately drawn to a woman about my age. She was exquisite. Stunning. I inwardly thought, *Wish I looked like that—she's so classy.* Later Marti sought me out. "Linda, I have to talk to you. I can't talk to anyone in our church or in this city. Please, can we get together?"

It is difficult to shock me, but what Marti told me made my mind whirl and my heart ache. She said, "My husband told me that he loved me, admired me, and wanted to be married to me, BUT that there was no chemistry anymore and there would be no sexual relationship. Most women wish their husbands had a headache occasionally, but mine has a perpetual headache."

Many women believe that any man would be overwhelmed with desire if he had a wife who looked like Marti, but this was not the case. During the weekend retreat, I talked with two other women whose husbands claimed disinterest in sex. Three women in one weekend? It seems husbands who are "cold fish" is a more common problem than women realize. Most women with this problem are too embarrassed to bring it up—especially when other wives are wishing their husbands weren't *so* interested in sex.

According to Dr. Janet Wolfe, author of *What to Do When He Has a Headache*, 50 to 60 percent of the time the complaint that one's partner has fizzled out sexually comes from a woman. In her book, Dr. Wolfe cites a *Redbook* magazine study of more than a hundred thousand married women that revealed almost four wives in ten, or 38 percent, felt they were not having sex often enough. These statistics indicate that increasingly today's marriage dilemma is, "My husband isn't interested."[1]

As you might imagine, this situation stirs up deep feelings of insecurity and doubt within these women:

> "I'm jealous of women whose husbands desire them."

> "I'm not sure why, but I feel ashamed."

> "I used to think I was attractive, but now I analyze everything I put on. I'm obsessed with my appearance."

> "I pick a fight before we go to bed. Then when he doesn't want to make love, I tell myself it's because of the argument."

> "I feel so vulnerable. I'm an affair waiting to happen."

> "I can't help but wonder where he's getting his sexual needs met. Is he into porn? Is there another woman?"

One woman wrote:

> The pain is so piercing. The core of my femininity has been crushed. I've worked at being an exciting lover to my husband, and what do I

get? Rejected. What is wrong with him? What is wrong with *me*? I know I don't look like Cindy Crawford, but everyone says I'm attractive. My husband makes me feel oversexed when all I want is a "normal" sexual relationship. I hate to approach him because I can't handle another "brush off." What does God want me to do with my sexuality? In my heart I long to be faithful to God and to my husband, but today I feel like running away. My thoughts scare me. I really think other men would find me a great lover. *God, keep me from thinking such things! I know I'm vulnerable to the attention of another man. I'm scared.*

The problem no one talks about is a *real* problem. What causes it?

IDENTIFYING THE PROBLEM

An expert in sexual issues made the following statement: "Ninety percent of sexual problems aren't sexual at all—they have their roots in the emotional barriers we place between ourselves and our partners. We bring these problems into the bedroom from the dinner table, the office, from our past experiences."[2] The reasons why a man may lack sexual interest include: changing sex roles, fear of closeness, feeling overworked and overstressed, time pressures, boredom, marital conflict, anger, and fear of sexual dysfunction.[3]

Does God's Word address this issue? Yes. Let's look at 1 Corinthians 7:3-5 (Message).

> Sexual drives are strong, but marriage is strong enough to contain them and provide for a balanced and fulfilling sexual life in a world of sexual disorder. The marriage bed must be a place of mutuality—the husband seeking to satisfy his wife, the wife seeking to satisfy her husband. Marriage is not a place to "stand up for your rights." Marriage is a decision to serve the other, whether in bed or out. Abstaining from sex is permissible for a period of time if you both agree to it, and if it's for the purposes of prayer and fasting—but only for such times. Then come back together again. Satan has an ingenious way of tempting us when we least expect it. I'm not, understand, commanding these periods of abstinence—only providing my best counsel if you should choose them.

These verses make it clear that:

- Celibacy is wrong for married couples. If your husband is pursuing a semi-celibate state, he is in sin because he is withholding what is rightly yours.
- Sexual expression between a husband and wife is not an option; it is part of our God-given responsibility to each other.
- Your husband doesn't have authority over his body—you do!
- The only reason to abstain from sex is prayer and fasting.

What do you do with this knowledge? Do you club your husband over the head and say, "God's Word says you're wrong!" Obviously that's not the best course of action. The best thing to do is to have an honest talk with God and then an honest talk with your husband.

AN HONEST TALK WITH GOD

> Search me, O God, and know my heart; try me and know my anxious thoughts; and see if there be any hurtful way in me, and lead me in the everlasting way. (Psalm 139:23-24)

Why does David ask God to search his heart? David was a diligent self-searcher yet could not see any wicked way in himself. He knew God was a better searcher so he invited God to dig into his heart. C. H. Spurgeon, in *The Treasury of David* calls this process "Divine scrutiny in order to be informed of errors and defects." [4] Are you willing for God to search your heart? Will you pray?

> *God, I've examined my heart—I'm not sure if there are wrong attitudes or actions (wickedness) but You see clearly. I invite You to search the innermost parts of my being and reveal any error in my thinking or in my ways. Have I tried to control my husband? Have I criticized him? Have I cut him down? Show me any "hurtful way" that might have caused him to turn from me sexually. Then, Lord, should You reveal any way in which I have failed You or my husband, give me the courage to do what is right to make amends.*

After you have honestly talked to God and asked Him to search your heart and reveal any sin in your life, it is time to talk to your husband.

AN HONEST TALK WITH YOUR HUSBAND

How do you talk honestly about sex when you've been so wounded by your husband? First and foremost, follow 1 Corinthians 16:14: "Let all that you do be done in love." (Can you imagine the difference it would make in our marriages if we consistently applied just that one verse!) Ephesians 4:15 commands us to speak "the truth in love." The key word is *love*. Often the truth is spoken—but in anger, not in love. Tell your husband exactly what you are feeling and how you are struggling, but make certain your communication is loving. Ask him if you have done anything (controlled, criticized, cut him down) to contribute to the problem of his lack of interest sexually.

It is very difficult to have this honest talk. How do you speak loving, truthful words, when all you feel is hurt? One woman's solution was to have the talk via a letter.

> Dear Toby,
>
> I am writing you because I love you and want our marriage to be the best it can be. I want to become the wife you need. I've tried many times to express to you in person what I'm feeling inside and it seems we always end up arguing, so I'm going to try writing this letter. I realize it is difficult for both of us to talk about these things. I really don't know why you've lost interest in me sexually, but I want to understand. I know I don't have a perfect body, but I'm not unattractive either. I'm scared, Toby, because I feel like our sexual relationship (really the lack of it) is changing the way we relate to each other. I feel unloved, unattractive, undesirable, and very vulnerable. A man complimented me at church Sunday, and I've thought about him all week. Please, will you talk to me and go with me for help? I want our marriage to work!

Whether or not you write your husband a letter or try talking openly to him is between you and God. God cares deeply about the sexual problem in your marriage. He is the One who can reveal to you how to relate to your husband in love. You are unique. Your sexual relationship is unique. Your marriage is unique. Each woman must decide for herself, with God's guidance, what is best for her marriage.

HOW CHRISTI HANDLED HER SITUATION

Christi, mother of two and married twelve years, said, "My husband and I didn't make love for a year. He had excuses that, at the time, seemed legitimate. I had tried to approach him sexually but was refused. It was hard to keep asking, but I realized that our lack of physical intimacy had seriously hurt our marriage. I thought, *What should I do? How do I get out of a 'no lovemaking rut'?*

"Finally I thought, *I've got to take the initiative again.* I asked my husband, 'What can I do to turn you on?' His answer sliced into me . . . 'Nothing.' But I tried everything I could think of anyway—a sexy nightie, creative seduction. You name it, I tried it. I even added mystery. I took him to each room of the house where a card gave him a clue as to where to go next. The final room was the bedroom (of course) where I served him dinner in bed. He was pleased with the gourmet meal and then made it clear he wanted to watch TV—he didn't want to make love to me. Only a woman who has been rejected knows the humiliation, the rage, the feeling of helplessness."

Christi told her husband how she felt, both verbally and in letters, but he just wouldn't talk about it. They also went to a Christian counselor, but there was no change. We wish we could tell you that Christi discovered a magical formula and now she and her husband enjoy passionate love three times a week. But that's not the case. Christi couldn't fix the problem, but she found a new way of looking at her situation that has helped her deal with the pain of her husband's rejection.

"I have realized that it is *his* problem, not mine," Christi says. "I came to the conclusion that I couldn't make choices for my husband, but I could be responsible for my actions. I made a commitment to the Lord to cling to Him, to turn my constant worries into prayers for our sexual relationship. I asked myself, 'What if the situation never changes?' I decided to live with an eternal perspective, with my eyes focused on Christ rather than on my hurt. My situation hasn't changed, but I'm more at peace."

Christi received comfort from 1 Peter 2:18–3:12. She wrote this paraphrase of the passage and has often prayed it to God, asking God to give her His perspective.

> *O God, thank You that when I love my unlovable husband, this finds favor with You. It is easier to love someone who is loving me, but I choose to follow in Christ's steps by loving even when I am rejected. It is so difficult, God. Only as You are my strength can I not insult back when I am insulted. I want to threaten and say ugly things but, Lord, You've asked me to trust everything—my feelings of rejection, my anger, my future—to You who judges justly. Show me, God, how to live my faith before my husband, how to "walk my talk" before him. I don't know what it looks like to return a blessing for an insult. Guide me, Holy God. I commit to refrain my tongue from speaking evil and seek peace with my husband. Thank You for Your promise that You will hear my prayer.*

Women whose husbands do not desire them sexually experience tremendous pain and frustration. There is another group of women who experience these same feelings, but with a slightly different slant.

MY HUSBAND WANTS ME BUT CAN'T . . .

These women have husbands who are interested in sex, but for some reason are unable to perform sexually. What prevents a man from being able to maintain an erection? Medication is a big culprit. Check what medications your husband is taking and ask your doctor or pharmacist about over-the-counter and prescription drugs (see page 126) as they can significantly decrease a person's interest in sex. Drugs that often inhibit sexual desire include antihistamines, antidepressants, antipsychotics, beta blockers, decongestants, and tranquilizers.[5]

When a man suddenly finds himself without a sex drive or impotent, whether due to medication or another reason, it can devastate him. Lana's husband was fifty when he began taking a medication for depression that dulled his sexual senses. He felt old and thought he'd lost his virility. He was distressed; so was Lana. Her femininity was threatened, and she was afraid. "Will he give in to some kind of temptation? Will he turn to pornography?" Her husband felt insecure. Lana felt insecure. They both feared being intimate, and lovemaking was avoided. But Lana prayed, *Lord, show me how to encourage him, how to affirm his manliness. God, don't let me fall into the trap of feeling he isn't attracted to me and take it personally. I ask You for restoration. Give me patience, and show me how to love this man. Give me wisdom to know how to build him up.*

As Lana waited on God, He gave wisdom and perspective to help them get through this difficult time. She did five things to improve their sexual relationship.

1. She gained insight about how her husband's sexual inabilities affected him. Lana began to understand that God created women's bodies in a way that continually affirms their femininity and sexuality. Every month, through PMS and having a period, she was reminded that she was a woman, feminine, created to bear children. She remembered carrying a baby in her womb, feeling the first flutters of movement within, then marveling at the miracle of birth. She nursed her child. Over and over, in myriad ways, her body shouted, "You are woman; you are feminine."

DRUGS THAT AFFECT SEXUALITY[6]

Category	Common Brand Name
ANTIHYPERTENSIVES Used to treat high blood pressure	Aldoclor, Aldomet, Inderal, Indride, Emelin, Diuperes, Hydropres, Minipress, Minizide, Catapres-TTS
ANTIDEPRESSANTS Used to treat depression	Tofranil, Desyrel, Nardil, Anafranil, Asendin, Prozac, Paxil, Zoloft, Elavil
ANTIANXIETY Used to treat anxiety	Xanax, Valium, Libritabs, Limbitrol
MISCELLANEOUS	Lanoxin, Norpace, Tagamet, Diamox, Proscar, Procardia, Zoladex

She pondered the ways God created a man's body to affirm his masculinity. A man's muscles, physical stamina, and physique all contribute to his masculinity, but the primary way masculinity is affirmed for a man is through his prowess as a lover. His sexual drive causes his erection and gives him the desire to woo his wife. It is impossible to express how much of a man's masculinity is tied up in his ability as a lover.

2. She broached the subject with her husband. Instead of ignoring the problem, hoping it would resolve itself, Lana boldly approached her husband and spoke these beautiful affirming words to him. "Honey, I'm here, I'm available, anytime. I love you, I want you. I loved our relationship when it was wildly physical like a roaring blaze, but I love it now when the fire is more of a cozy warmth."

3. She built up his masculinity. Lana told us, "I became much more intentional in affirming my husband's qualities as a leader. I admired his spiritual power, his diligent work, his protection of me, and provision for me. I told him of the respect his children had for him. Through words and tender touch, I admired his character as well as his body."

4. She encouraged her husband to find an alternative to the medication he was taking. Lana scheduled a second honeymoon in California to foster romantic moments. While she and her husband were there, they met with a nutrition specialist. "Together, we implemented a new eating plan that would allow my husband to go off his medication. Slowly, his sexual function is returning."

5. Lana trusted God to meet her needs. Lana realized she had depended too much upon her husband to meet her needs. She came to realize that by doing this, she had placed unfair expectations upon him and set herself up for disappointment. "Only God can meet my needs. When I give my needs to Him, He often meets them in the most unexpected ways. I thank Him for this trial in our marriage because it forced me to rely more heavily upon God. He has become my Rock and Refuge, my Hope and my Help."

Lana sought God and was proactive in reaching out to her husband. Your husband may be thirty and uninterested in sex for reasons only God knows. He may be fifty and suffering the affects of medication or illness, or he may have had radical prostate surgery and sexual function seems forever lost. Whatever your situation, you are probably asking, "What can I do?"

Help for You

Women have asked us, "How do I handle my sexuality when my husband isn't interested or is not able to function sexually?" First and foremost, stay close to the Lord and seek His perspective. God has allowed this in your life, therefore God promises to work character, perseverance, and hope in your life as you turn to Him (Romans 5:3-5).

Second, stay busy and occupied with thinking about others and not yourself. Become active physically: jogging, walking, or swimming. This proved very helpful for Katelyn who reports: "God made it clear to me that until something changes in my marriage, I am to live like a nun. I often take cold showers and rechannel sexual energy through brisk walks. (I think I've walked around the globe twice now.) I know that God is able to sustain me. I am at peace with this present course."

Other women have asked us point-blank, "If my husband can't (or won't) satisfy me sexually, is it okay for me to satisfy myself?" As we stated in the introduction, in preparation for writing this book we read through the Bible from Genesis to Revelation and noted every verse pertaining to the sexual relationship. Concerning self-pleasuring, the Scriptures are silent, saying that such actions are neither right or wrong. Some Christians denounce masturbation based on the story of Onan in Genesis 38, but theologian and sex therapist Dr. Douglas Rosenau says this is a gross misinterpretation of the Genesis account.[7]

Some women feel self-pleasuring in certain circumstances is allowed based on verses such as, "I know and am convinced in the Lord Jesus that nothing is unclean in itself; but to him who thinks anything to be unclean, to him it is unclean" (Romans 14:14). In response to this, Dr. Rosenau quotes 1 Corinthians 6:12: "All things are lawful for me, but all things are not helpful. All things are lawful for me, *but I will not be brought under the power of any*" (NKJV, emphasis ours). Under certain circumstances, Dr. Rosenau says self-pleasuring is permissible but adds this warning. Any sexual behavior that becomes a habit can be detrimental to and narrow your sex life. In any type of sexual pleasuring, especially self-pleasuring, you must guard your fantasy and thought life . . . and not have your partnership adulterated by fantasizing about other people. This point is vital if you use self-pleasuring as a solitary activity to release sexual tension.[8]

In *The Gift of Sex,* Clifford and Joyce Penner suggest that a man or woman ask themselves if self-stimulation is loving. "If one partner desires a great deal of sexual activity and the other is less frequently interested, the couple might decide that masturbation is the most loving act the highly interested person can do."[9]

Many Christian books, like Rosenau's and the Penners', give helpful information about this sensitive topic, but ultimately as we have said, each woman must go to God and seek Him. Only God can clarify when the Scriptures are silent. This is a very personal issue, one in which you need His guidance. Ask Him what is right and appropriate for you in your situation.

GUARD YOUR HEART

If you are in a marriage where your husband is disinterested in sex or unable to be interested, you must guard your heart, your eyes, and your activities. Some Christian women who would never look at pornographic literature or watch an X-rated video spend hours lost in romance novels. They watch movies and fantasize about other men who would "romance" them as they deserve and be the lover of their dreams.

Escaping into steamy novels for a woman is similar to a man escaping into pornography. Both are seeking to live in a fantasy world.

Other women send sexual signals to men who show an interest in them in order to reaffirm their sexuality. They dismiss their actions as harmless flirtation, when in reality, they are placing themselves in a precarious situation. If you fall into this category, we encourage you to read chapter 9 about how to handle sexual temptation. Dear friend, set a guard around your heart, your eyes, and your activities.

HELP FOR HUBBY

1. Physiological help. As we write, the new drug Viagra has just become available. A cover story in *USA Today* reads, "Doctors tout wonders of the little pill that could. Taken an hour before intercourse, Viagra works on normal body chemistry to allow blood to rush into the penis when a man is sexually stimulated."[10] The hope is that Viagra will prove to be a pill with potential for male performance, but at this time, the jury is still out.[11] (There is concern about potential side effects and combining Viagra with other medications.) Many are excited about its possibilities while others look for natural helps. They ask, "Is there such a thing as an aphrodisiac?"

All kinds of food, drug, or drink has at one time or another been used to call forth sexual desire—from substances as ordinary as an apple to those as strange as hippopotamus snout. Although the Food and Drug Administration says there is no over-the-counter food, lotion, potion, or medication that fits the bill as an aphrodisiac, others argue that there are some substances that really do arouse sexuality.[12]

The ancient Chinese belief that ginseng is a mild sexual stimulant is accepted by some. Herb companies market ginseng teas, capsules, tablets, and tinctures. One way to enjoy ginseng is as a refreshing tea. Add one-half teaspoon of powdered root per cup of boiling water. Simmer ten minutes. Then drink hot or cold. To add more flavor, try honey and lemon or mix with a flavored tea.[13]

According to herbalist, Diana De Luca, author of *Botanica Erotica,* another help is oats. Have you heard, "The horse is feeling its oats" or "The young man is sowing his wild oats"? Ever wonder what oats had to do with sexuality? De Luca suggests eating oatmeal to stimulate sexual interest. (Your mother was right; oatmeal is good for you.) She also suggests a specially blended tea to help in this area. To brew the tea, steep two big teaspoons of oats or green oat straw overnight (purchase at a health food store), then drink the tea warm the next day. Who knows, your husband might start "feeling his wild oats"!

There is one natural aphrodisiac—and it's not oysters, chocolate, or ginseng—but exercise. Cardiovascular fitness seems to have a direct effect on men's sexual performance because attaining and maintaining an erection requires good circulation. And one of the body's responses to regular exercise is increased blood volume throughout the entire body. Several studies have shown that testosterone levels rise after short-term moderately vigorous exercise.[14]

Perhaps two ways you could help your husband would be to invite him for a walk with you each evening or give both of you a membership to a gym and begin working out together. After your exercise time, indulge in a cooling glass of ginseng tea!

2. Spiritual help. Exercise and a positive attitude will help you and your husband as you struggle through his lack of interest or ability sexually. But the greatest help will be found on your knees. Let us ask you a question. When was the last time you prayed about the problems in your sexual relationship? You've been frustrated, hurt, and angry, but have you prayed? God is very concerned about your marriage, including your sexual relationship. Fall on your knees before Him, pour out your heart, your hurt to Him. Ask Him to show you how to love your husband, how to affirm him, how to encourage him in his masculinity. Ask God specifically if there is anything you can do to create desire in your man.

God weeps with you. Ask Him to carry you when you can't walk, and thank Him that in HIM, *there is hope.*

The prophet Jeremiah wept before the Lord, "My soul has been rejected from peace; I have forgotten happiness. So I say, 'My strength has perished, and so has my hope from the LORD'" (Lamentations 3:17-18). But Jeremiah refused to remain in this hopeless state. He shifted his focus from his pain and unhappiness to his eternal, loving God. May you do the same and regain hope.

> This I recall to mind and therefore I have hope. The lovingkindness of the LORD never ceases, His mercies are new every morning. Great is Thy faithfulness. "The LORD is my portion," says my soul, "therefore I will hope in Him." (Lamentations 3:21-24, our paraphrase)

CHANGE MY HEART, O GOD

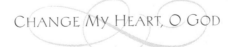

1. Lana initiated a five-step program, pages 126-7 to help her sexual relationship with her husband. Develop your own plan of action. Incorporate some of Lana's steps or devise your own.

2. Memorize Lamentations 3:21-24, and pray it back to God.

COMMUNICATION DOS AND DON'TS

Don't say to him:

- ❧ "I thought men loved sex; what is wrong with you?"
- ❧ "Denise's husband wants to make love continually."
- ❧ "If we're going to live as roommates, I'm out of here."

Don't say to yourself:

- ❧ "I'm not attractive."
- ❧ "This must be my problem."
- ❧ "There is no hope."

Do say to him:

- ❧ "I love you just the way you are."
- ❧ "I am committed to you."
- ❧ "There's no one I'd rather be with than you."

Do say to yourself:

- ❧ "I am beautiful, a precious gem in God's eyes."
- ❧ "I will lift my husband up to God and pray for this area of his life."
- ❧ "Nothing is impossible with God." (Jeremiah 32:17)

twelve

How Can I Get Rid of Guilt
over My Abortion?

From the moment the dentist had turned on the drill, Maryanne hadn't been able to stop crying. *What is wrong with me?* she thought. *I'm not in pain. There's enough Novocaine in me to numb a rhinoceros.*

"I'm sorry," she apologized later. "I don't know why the drill made me cry. I certainly wasn't abused as a child or anything!" They both laughed awkwardly, each certain the drill had triggered something deep within her, but neither knowing what.

This crying episode haunted Maryanne for several years. Then one day she read an article that said that women who suffer from post-abortion syndrome often weep when they hear the sound of a dentist's drill because it reminds them of the high-pitched whine of the vacuum used in abortion clinics.

When she was nineteen and unmarried, Maryanne discovered she was pregnant. She spent little time analyzing her situation. The pregnancy was a problem, and the way to fix the problem was to eliminate it. In those days, there were no pro-life activists waving pictures of aborted fetuses, no people handing out literature outside the clinic in an effort to save babies. It was only later—ten years later—that Maryanne acknowledged that what she had aborted from her womb had been a living child.

She had asked God to forgive her, but instead of feeling forgiven, Maryanne felt guilty. She'd squirmed uncomfortably in her seat when her pastor had urged the congregation to participate in a right-to-life march. Each time her best friend—a strong pro-life activist—passionately condemned the suffering of unborn babies, she felt as if a knife had pierced her heart. The pro-life bumper sticker on her neighbor's Toyota pointed an accusing finger in her face, "You murderer." Even her own children aroused her guilt!

As she watched them grow, she couldn't help wondering what her unborn child might have been like. Each year on the anniversary of "the deed," she mentally advanced the child's age and speculated how he might have fit into her existing family if he had lived.

No one knew about the abortion except the friend who had driven her home from the clinic. She'd never even told her husband because, after all, that was in the past. But if the abortion was in the past, why was the present becoming a living hell?

IF ONLY I COULD FORGET

In the past twenty-five years since the U.S. Supreme Court legalized unrestricted abortion, approximately thirty-seven million abortions have occurred.[1] Some, like Maryanne, abort because a baby doesn't fit into their plans or their husband's plans. Others seek an abortion because they are pressured by uncommitted boyfriends or by parents who don't want to shame the family name. A few abort because impregnation was forced upon them, and they want everything connected with that violent act removed from their lives.

Though the reasons differ, nearly every woman has the same emotion when she walks out of an abortion clinic: "I want to put this behind me and get on with my life." At first, a woman may believe she has succeeded in this goal, but over time emotions associated with the abortion surface. Instead of acknowledging these emotions, she stuffs them down and snaps on a lid labeled "things to forget." But a woman who has had an abortion can never forget. Forgetting only serves to temporarily numb the pain; to be healed, she must remember.

Dr. Paul Reisser and his wife Teri, who have counseled hundreds of women with post-abortion syndrome (PAS), say, "The very first task of healing is for the woman to access the negative feelings that surrounded the abortion experience. Most women have utilized repression as a coping strategy for so long that they have long forgotten the fear, anger, guilt, and grief associated with the abortion. Until these powerful emotions are fresh in the woman's mind again, there is literally not much with which to work."[2]

Most women who go through an abortion deny the experience on one of three levels:

1. Deny the act: Some women assuage guilt by excusing the act of abortion with comments such as, "Abortion is legal" (translation: abortion is okay) and "It's my body, I can do what I want."

2. Deny the fact: A Christian who has had an abortion feels conflict in her spirit between the truth of God's Word—life begins at conception—and her decision to abort. God's Word reminds her: "For you created my inmost being; you knit me together in my mother's womb . . . your eyes saw my unformed body. All the days ordained for me were written in your book before one of them came to be" (Psalm 139:13,16, NIV). Yet this woman pacifies her inner conflict by deceiving herself into believing, "It was only a glob of tissue, not a real baby."

3. Deny the impact: Many who have had abortions try to sidestep guilt by convincing themselves, "It was years ago. It shouldn't matter today." Or, "Sex with my husband is less than terrific, but I'm sure this has no connection to my abortion."

Denying the act, the fact, and the impact are attempts to avoid facing what we have done. As long as we cover up, hide, excuse, and rationalize, the guilt of abortion will haunt us. If we want to be healed, we must remember what happened. Yes, remembering hurts. But it is necessary to move toward healing.

Are you brave enough to remove the lid from the emotions you've sealed off? We know it's scary. But for healing to occur, you must admit your hurt, remove the infection, and then flood the wound with fresh water and allow it to heal.

We understand your reluctance to relive these memories, but the longer you wait, the more painful it will be. Before going any further, why don't you stop and pray? Inviting God to be with you will give you the strength you need to take this important step.

Father, I don't want to remember. It's easier to convince myself that it doesn't matter, that what I did was no big deal. God, in my heart I

know that's a lie! What I did grieved You. It grieved others. It grieves
me. The ache in my soul will never go away until I fully lay my abor-
tion and my unborn child before you. I'm scared, but I can do this
knowing You are with me. If it takes "going back" to go forward, I
am willing.

We encourage you NOT to read on until this prayer is the cry of your
heart. Then, when you are ready, when you sense God's presence and feel
His strength with you, go forward in healing.

FOUR STEPS TO HEALING

Healing from abortion generally involves four steps: remembering, asking
forgiveness, accepting forgiveness, and releasing your unborn child into
God's care.

Maryanne followed these steps and God healed her. In order to better
understand how this process works, we will walk you through each step
using Maryanne as an example. As you read, ask God to work in your heart
and to heal your hurt.

1. Remembering. "He who conceals his sins does not prosper, but who-
ever confesses and renounces them finds mercy" (Proverbs 28:13, NIV).

Maryanne had concealed her abortion from those who loved her most;
her husband, her family, and her close friends. The black hole of secrecy
eroded her normally cheerful countenance and she became depressed and
listless. Sex with her husband was emotionless and mechanical, partly
because she emotionally held him at arm's length for fear he would discover
what she'd done and partly because sex before marriage had been the vehicle
for great suffering.

After reading the article that explained her reaction to the dentist's drill,
Maryanne realized she was suffering from post-abortion syndrome.
Healing, the article said, began with remembering. Even though every
emotion in her screamed against it, for the sake of herself and for the sake
of her loved ones, she would force herself to remember.

Maryanne remembered the shock she felt at the doctor's announcement
that she was pregnant. She and her boyfriend had had sex only three times.

Knowing she was not married, the doctor handed Maryanne a card with the name of a counselor at a local "woman's center" [abortion clinic]. Mechanically, she reached for the card and used the phone in his office to make an appointment.

The following morning Maryanne bombarded the counselor with questions. Would the procedure hurt? What was involved? How long would it take? What were the risks? The counselor had answers for every question except for the one that troubled her most: Why was this happening to her?

On Saturday, she joined twenty other women in the waiting room of the clinic. She hung her head, avoiding eye contact. She knew none of these women, yet she felt an odd sense of kinship with these strangers who shared her fate. Maryanne recalls:

> An unsmiling nurse called my number. She ushered me into a room and instructed me to slip into a formless gown. Minutes later, she guided me to another room, pointed to an operating bed and told me to lie down. As she injected me full of pain-numbing drugs, I studied the table on my right which displayed the sterilized instruments the doctor would use inside me. The room spun. Objects blurred. I was in a nightmare from which I couldn't escape. I heard the whirring of the vacuum, felt a tugging sensation in my uterus, sensed the pressure of the nurse's hand on my abdomen. Then I blacked out.
>
> The next thing I remember was lying on a hard, flat bed in a small room with three other women. We were told: "Drink the juice. Eat the crackers. Rest for thirty minutes." I glanced at the young girl lying on the bed next to mine. What was she thinking? Did she feel as though she had just committed an evil sin? Or was she relieved that her "situation" had been taken care of? Did she feel a sense of loss? My own sense of loss was profound, but I could not name the loss, nor could I say exactly what had been taken from me.

Maryanne wept for hours after reliving these memories, but in her weeping she confronted the truth. It had taken ten years, but she finally acknowledged that what had been taken from her had been a baby. *Her* baby.

2. Asking forgiveness. "For the sake of your name, O LORD, forgive my iniquity, though it is great" (Psalm 25:11, NIV).

A month after Maryanne had taken the first step of remembering, the director of the Crisis Pregnancy program showed a film at her Sunday school class. The film depicted an eight-week-old fetus in the womb. The hands, feet, and eyes of the baby were clearly visible. The images unsettled her as she had aborted her child at eight weeks of age. The baby's tiny hand jerked up and down as if waving, "Hi, Mommy."

At home, Maryanne locked herself in her bedroom and prayed:

> Oh, Lord, I am a sinner! I ignored Your command to save myself for marriage. Then, when I found out I was pregnant, I added sin upon sin by delivering my child to an abortionist to be killed. Oh, God! How could I have callously destroyed my child? It wasn't just my child that I hurt. I hurt others: my boyfriend, my parents, the friends I pushed away for fear they would find out what I had done and hate me, and my husband. I hurt him by not trusting him and by keeping him in the dark about why sex isn't all that fun for me. Most of all, God, I hurt You. I disobeyed You, disappointed You, distanced myself from You. I accused You of being distant, but I'm the one who kept us from being close. I was too ashamed to come into Your presence. Forgive me, Lord. Forgive the blood on my hands and sin in my heart.

No matter how great our sin, God stands ready to forgive. His Word is clear: "If we confess our sins, he is faithful and just and will forgive us our sins and purify us from all unrighteousness" (1 John 1:9, NIV). But confessing is only the first step in receiving forgiveness. If we want to be healed, we must go a step further and receive the forgiveness God offers.

3. Accepting forgiveness. "If you, O LORD, kept a record of sins, O Lord, who could stand? But with you there is forgiveness" (Psalm 130:3-4, NIV).

It is often easier to ask for forgiveness than to receive it. Shame reminds us that we are unworthy sinners. Guilt convicts us of our wickedness. Satan mocks us with thoughts like, "What would a holy God want with the likes of you?"

Maryanne knew she was unworthy to receive forgiveness but she resisted the temptation to short-circuit healing by giving in to guilt and shame. By faith, she reached out and took the gift God offered. Maryanne shares:

> What happened next was like nothing I had ever experienced before— or since. I felt what I can only describe as a white waterfall pour over me. It was warm, with water and light all mixed together. Though I couldn't see its source, I knew it flowed from the throne of God. I felt free! Clean and forgiven. I wanted to laugh, to dance, to sing. I stood up, lifted my arms to heaven and joyously soaked in the presence of the Holy One who poured out His grace upon me.

In chapter 8, we talked about David's experience of God's forgiveness after he confessed to committing adultery and murder. Like Maryanne, he exulted in knowing he was forgiven. In Psalm 42:7-8 (NIV) he says: "Deep calls to deep in the roar of your waterfalls; all your waves and breakers have swept over me. By day the LORD directs his love, at night his song is with me."

After receiving God's forgiveness, Maryanne spent a great deal of time in prayer extending that same forgiveness to others. She forgave her boyfriend for abandoning her, she forgave her parents for their blindness to her misery, she forgave insensitive comments made by people at church about "baby killers." And, she asked her husband to forgive her for her failure to trust him with her secret.

Forgiveness, like the rushing waterfall, cannot be contained. It spills over into every crevice in our lives, then flows out healing and love to others.

4. Releasing your child to God. "Let the little children come to me, and do not hinder them, for the kingdom of God belongs to such as these" (Mark 10:14, NIV).

God pronounced Maryanne clean and blameless based on her acceptance of Christ's payment for her sin. But for her healing to be complete, Maryanne needed to take a final step; she needed to release her child into the care of God.

Releasing a child into God's care is not about following prescribed actions, rather it is an acknowledgement in a woman's heart that her child was real, that God cares about the child and will watch over him or her. For some women, releasing a child into God's care might be a simple prayer acknowledging the baby and seeing that baby under the protection of her heavenly Father. For others, it might involve mentally assenting with the beautiful image in the poem "The Babe I'll Never Hold" (see page 141).

Maryanne found it helpful to do something concrete, like naming her baby and holding a memorial service.

Maryanne believed her child was a girl. She named her Tina ("tiny one"). She asked her husband, pastor, and several close friends if they would attend a short memorial service in Tina's honor. They agreed. It was a powerful experience for Maryanne. She told us:

> The service was held in the garden in my backyard. My pastor read from Psalm 23: "The LORD is my shepherd: I shall not want. . . . Surely goodness and mercy shall follow me all the days of my life; . . . I will dwell in the house of the LORD forever." As he read, I pictured Tina in my arms. We walked through green pastures and by still waters. Tina cooed with delight as I traced the contours of her face. God called her name. It was time to let go. I lifted my arms upward. God reached out and took hold of my daughter. My empty arms ached, but I knew everything would be okay. My last image of Tina was of her in the arms of God. Her tiny hand was waving, "Bye, Mommy." I waved back and whispered, "Good-bye, Tina. One day we will be together again."
>
> We planted a small oak tree in the center of the garden in memory of Tina and then shared communion. Afterwards, we each filled our communion cups with water and poured it out on the tree. Each time I look out my kitchen window and see the tree, I am reminded that Tina is not dead, she is alive and safe in the arms of God.

Releasing your child into God's care is not part of receiving forgiveness. If you have followed the first two steps, your forgiveness is complete. But your healing may not be. Releasing your child to God promotes healing and places mental and emotional closure on your hurt. As you pray and weep through this step, God will heal. "I have heard your prayer and seen your tears; I will heal you" (2 Kings 20:5, NIV).

BEAUTY FROM ASHES

Today, Maryanne is healed from the guilt of her abortion. She often speaks at churches, sharing hope with others that no matter how great their sin, God can forgive and heal.

Another area God healed was Maryanne's sexual relationship with her husband, Ed. For years, the shame of her secret acted like an invisible wall between the two of them. Once the secret was disclosed, the wall came down and their physical relationship grew into something neither of them had thought possible. In the intimacy of lovemaking, Ed offered tender comfort to Maryanne.

THE BABE I'LL NEVER HOLD

If I knew then
   What I know now,
   You never would have died.
I'd have held you close
   And nurtured you
   And kept you by my side.
I'd have sung you songs
   And treasured you
   More than silver,
   More than gold:
But this song is all I'll give
To the Babe I'll never hold.

I've never written poetry
   That hasn't been a praise
To the Lord Who wept with me
   And held me through those days.
Jesus, now I'm asking.
   I know you hear my plea.
Won't you take that child in your hands
   And hold my Babe for me.[3]

—Anonymous

In Maryanne's life, God brought beauty out of ashes. He took what could be considered a curse and turned it into a blessing (Deuteronomy 23:5). He took her sin and used it to bring glory to His name. What happened for Maryanne can happen for you as well.

Do you believe this? Perhaps you think, *I want that. I do! But you said the first step in healing is to remember. The thought of reliving my past overwhelms me.*

Listen to what God says in response to such thoughts:

> Beloved, when you pass through the rivers, they will not sweep over you. When you walk through the fire, you will not be burned. For I, the Lord, will be with you. (See Isaiah 43:2-5.)

God promises to be with you, every step of the way:

> I will go before you and behind you. I will never leave you or forsake you. (See Deuteronomy 31:8, Isaiah 30:21.)

Don't worry about how long it will take . . . hold fast to His promises. God declares:

> The times and the seasons are mine to determine. I will give you new mercies each morning. When you are weak, I will be your strength. I will never give you more than you can bear. Trust me. (See Ecclesiastes 3:1, Lamentations 3:22-24, 1 Corinthians 10:13.)

> You are my precious child. I have great and wonderful plans for you, plans you could not imagine even if I told them to you now. (See Jeremiah 29:11.)

> Go forward, beloved. Go forward and be healed. (See Psalm 30:2.)

CHANGE MY HEART, O GOD

1. If you feel guilt over your abortion, pray the prayer at the beginning of the chapter on pages 135-6 and go through the four steps of healing. You will know you have been healed when you can say yes to each of these questions:

    - ❧ I believe what I did was a sin and I accept responsibility for my actions.
    - ❧ I have forgiven everyone connected with the abortion for their part in it, including myself.
    - ❧ I know what I aborted was not just a mass of tissue, but my living child.
    - ❧ I have received God's forgiveness for my sin.
    - ❧ I look forward to being reunited with my child.
    - ❧ I am able to talk about the abortion when it is appropriate to do so.

2. The fourth step, releasing your unborn child to God, is a step of closure and healing. For some women, it is enough simply to say a prayer of relinquishment. For others, a significant action or event, such as a memorial service, is helpful. Ask God what you need. If you feel He is leading you to do something concrete, consider writing a letter to your unborn child. Tell your child why you did what you did and how sorry you are. Tell your child the name you might have given him (or her). Describe some things you might have done together. Express your love and how you anticipate seeing your little one some day, but that for now it brings you joy to know he (or she) is safe in the arms of Jesus.

3. Memorize Jeremiah 29:11 (NIV): "'I know the plans I have for you,' declares the LORD, 'plans to prosper you and not to harm you, plans to give you hope and a future.'" As you memorize, praise God for what he has planned for you.

4. Review the resource material at the end of the chapter and prayerfully consider whether or not to seek out additional resources.

A WORD TO THE CHURCH

The pro-life movement has done an excellent job disseminating information on the evils of abortion. Christian media and right-to-life marches have increased awareness about the horrible genocide of babies. Each year thousands of churches participate in Sanctity of Life Sunday in which congregations are educated about the tragedy of abortion. Roses are distributed in memory of the babies who have died.

Such efforts should be applauded. Abortion *is* a tragedy, but it is also a tragedy if we, as the body of Christ, do not marry the message of the sin with the hope of forgiveness.

It is estimated that one in six women sitting in our churches has experienced an abortion.[4] Try to trade places, mentally, with one of these women, and imagine how she feels as she listens to impassioned pro-life speeches. The message of life can become a message of death when it is not tempered with grace. Pray for God to show you how you can be an instrument of healing to the silent wounded in your church.

A WORD ABOUT POST-ABORTION SYNDROME

Ninety-four percent of women admit experiencing negative psychological effects following an abortion.[5] Post-abortion syndrome (PAS) is a term that describes a woman's inability to (1) process the fear, anger, sadness, and guilt surrounding her abortion experience, (2) grieve the loss of her baby, and (3) come to peace with God, herself, and others involved in the abortion decision.[6] Following are some of the actions and emotions often associated with a woman suffering from PAS:

Guilt. Post-abortion women suffering from extreme guilt tend to beat themselves up emotionally, punish themselves, or unjustly condemn themselves. They believe if something bad happens, it is because they deserve it. Such guilt often leads to abnormal behaviors.

Self-destructive behaviors. Self-destructive behaviors include becoming involved in an abusive relationship, promiscuity, drug and alcohol abuse, suicide attempts, eating disorders, and workaholism.

Anxiety. This includes irritability, inability to relax, dizziness, pounding heart, upset stomach, headaches, inconsistent sleep patterns, inability to concentrate, and extreme duress about the future. Prolonged anxiety can lead to panic attacks and irrational fears. Very often a woman with PAS will not relate her anxiety to her abortion, and yet she will unconsciously begin to avoid anything having to do with babies (showers, the baby aisle at the grocery store, etc.).[7]

Emotional numbness. To avoid facing the emotional pain of aborting her child, a woman may make a conscious decision not to place herself in such a vulnerable situation again. Such a woman holds others at arm's length and avoids intimate relationships.

Depression. This includes feelings of overwhelming sadness, hopelessness, and despair which often result in sudden and uncontrollable crying episodes. Emotions can range from extreme anger to thoughts of suicide. Such thoughts frequently intensify around anniversary dates associated with the abortion.

Eating disorders. Because the post-abortion woman feels she lost control in becoming pregnant, she will sometimes become obsessive in controlling other areas of her life, such as food. Other times a woman will gain weight, subconsciously reasoning this will make her less attractive to men, and therefore less likely to be put in a position of aborting again.

Reduced motivation. Loss of enthusiasm for everyday living and reduced interest in pursuing meaningful relationships is common among PAS sufferers.

Flashbacks. Unusual responses to common experiences sometimes happen as the PAS sufferer relives her abortion experience. For example, the sound of a vacuum or a dentist drill can take her back to the vacuum used at abortion clinics. Certain sights, sounds, or smells may upset her. Sometimes women are troubled by nightmares that involve children screaming or situations in which they feel helpless.

Diminished interest in sex. PAS sufferers often punish themselves by refusing to give themselves permission to enjoy sex. They subconsciously feel that since sex was the prelude to the abortion, sexual activity should be avoided.

Preoccupation with becoming pregnant. Many PAS sufferers desire an "atonement baby" to replace the one that was lost and become obsessed with getting pregnant.

Where can you get more help?

See pages 257-8 for resources of organizations, Bible studies, books, and videos that address this subject.

thirteen

My Husband Is into Pornography—
What Should I Do?

*T*he caller refused to identify herself.

"Lorraine, I can't tell you my name, but I took part in a survey for the book you are writing with Linda Dillow."

"Yes . . .," I prompted, expecting her to continue. Instead, muffled sobs filtered through the receiver.

"Tell me what's wrong," I urged.

"It's my husband. I found a stack of pornographic magazines and videos in a closet in the garage. I knew he'd had a problem with pornography when he was a boy, but he swore he was over it. Now he admits he's been looking at this junk off and on for the last five years!"

"Does anyone else know about this?" I asked.

"No. He's a leader in our church. He'd die if anyone found out."

"How do you feel about what he is doing?"

"One minute I'm so disgusted I feel like throwing up. The next minute I want to strangle the life out of him. What is he thinking? How could he do this to me?" She paused. The rage storming within her gathered force and exploded in one, heart-wrenching wail: "What's wrong with me that he would even want to look at pictures of other women?"

I let her cry, praying the tears would release the toxic emotions fuming inside her. A few minutes later she said she felt better. Like a violent tornado, her anger had swirled on, leaving behind the rubble of hopelessness and despair. "What shall I do?" she cried.

Discovering that your husband is into pornography is like being in a boxing ring with every negative emotion you've ever had. Anger, embarrassment, shock, shame, disgust—and all their nasty cousins—take turns punching and slugging you, until you crumple to the floor in a heap. Even when you are down, they continue to pummel you. Pain clouds your vision. You can't see which emotion hit you last, nor do you care. You only know you want the beating to stop. And like the anonymous caller, you believe the way to make it stop is to DO something.

But before you DO anything, you must first THINK something. Pornography is a battle for the mind and must be won in the mind. Perhaps you believe we are referring to your husband's mind. We are. But we are also talking about your mind. Your husband's use of pornography greatly affects you. Before you can help him, you must make sure your own thinking is right.

PORNOGRAPHY: A BATTLE FOR THE MIND

What do you think about yourself when you envision your husband studying some nameless woman's naked body? Do you question your femininity, your sexuality? Does your mind scream, *What's wrong with me? Am I really so terrible to look at?* Do you muse, *If only I had a forty-inch chest and long, shapely legs like the model in the magazine, he'd never look anywhere else?*

What do you feel when your mind accuses, *It's your fault your husband uses pornography* or when a "helpful" friend suggests, "He wouldn't need that stuff if you were a more skillful lover"?

Neal Clement, director of the American Family Associations OutReach Division, says, "You can't imagine how many times I've heard from a wife that she was told, 'You need to perform sexually for him.' This kind of advice is abusive. It makes a woman feel like the answer to his problem lies in her ability to bring him sexual gratification. This is just setting her up for a lot more hurt. It doesn't work and she's left feeling more shame and guilt because she couldn't do it for him."[1] One wife said, "I was victimized by well-meaning pastors. They told me, 'You're not satisfying your husband; you're not being a submissive wife.'"[2]

Friend, be aware. *Emotions associated with pornography don't fight fair.* If you are going to duke it out in your mind with your emotions, the only way you are going to win is if you set up two "boxing" rules.

Rule One: No comparing yourself with other women. The Bible calls the practice of comparing ourselves with others unwise (2 Corinthians 10:12). If we are comparing ourselves with images shown in pornography, perhaps a better word would be *absurd.* No one looks like those models. You don't. We don't. And, thanks to electronic editing, neither does the model! (A click of the mouse can zap the cottage cheese from her thighs or enlarge her breasts.)

Does this mean because we will never look like "that," we should abort all attempts to make our bodies and ourselves attractive for our husbands? No. As we discussed in chapter 6, our bodies are a temple of the Holy Spirit: We have a responsibility to be good stewards of what God has entrusted to us. We should eat right, exercise, discover dressing, makeup, and hairstyles that honor God and please our husbands. But we should never hold up the *Playboy* bunny or the *Victoria's Secret* model as a standard for beauty. To do so makes a mockery of God's prescription for feminine sexuality.

Rule Two: No condemning yourself. In *An Affair of the Mind,* Laurie Hall says, "A husband will work hard at convincing his wife and others that the addiction [to pornography] is her fault."[3] He does this to assuage his own guilt, but don't subscribe to such thinking. Beating yourself up is pointless and nonproductive. It also invites self-pity and therefore sin. "There is therefore now no condemnation for those who are in Christ Jesus" (Romans 8:1).

God does not want us to condemn ourselves. Neither does He want us to deceive ourselves into thinking we are perfect. We should always be open to correction and change, but God's way of achieving transformation is through loving instruction, not brutal condemnation.

How are you doing with the battle in your mind? Are you refusing to "compare" and "condemn?" Are you thinking right? If so, you are free to begin "doing." The first item on the to-do list is to increase your understanding of pornography and its dangers.

PORNOGRAPHY: BIG BUSINESS

Derived from the word *pornea*, which means sexually immoral, pornography is defined as words or graphic images intended to excite lascivious or lustful, lewd feelings. Before the introduction of *Playboy* magazine in 1954, pornography was a small business conducted in back alleys or through private sources. Today pornography is a booming eight- to thirteen-billion-dollar-a-year industry—that's more than the combined annual revenues for Coca Cola and McDonald-Douglas Corporation.[4] There are more outlets for pornography than there are Burger King restaurants ("Have it your way," the industry sings as the cash register rings.)

Three of the fastest growing markets are videos, the Internet, and phone sex.

In 1990, over 300 million X-rated videos were distributed in our neighborhoods—more than one sexually explicit video for every man, woman, and child living in our country.[5] The U.S. is the world's largest producer of adult movies, "churning out hard core videos at the astonishing rate of about 150 new titles a week."[6]

Computer users can log on to an estimated 72,000 pornographic websites where they can choose from a pornographic buffet of sexually explicit material.[7] These sites offer everything from pictures of couples engaged in oral sex to digital stripping. One of the most popular websites has 55,000 members and 250,000 visits daily from curious browsers who can view over 10,000 sexually explicit images.[8]

Between the hours of 9 P.M. and 1 A.M., nearly one quarter of a million people pick up the phone and dial up commercial phone sex. The average call lasts from six to eight minutes and ranges in cost from eighty-nine cents to four dollars a minute, netting phone-sex companies anywhere from $750 million to $1 billion a year.

But surely Christian men are not caught up in pornography, are they? Apparently so. Several weeks ago we brought up the subject in a Bible study group of ten women. Three of the ten shared that pornography was currently a factor in their marriage. Surveys conducted by the Christian organization, Promise Keepers, reveals that pornography is a widespread and growing problem.

The industry picture is shocking, but even more unsettling is the harmful impact pornography can have on the user.

DANGERS OF PORNOGRAPHY

The dangers of pornography are varied and numerous.

Pornography dehumanizes men and women. One wife said it well, "Pornography makes women feel used and men controlled." Debra Evans, author of *The Christian Woman's Guide to Sexuality,* agrees. "Erotica and porn depersonalize sex by removing it from the purpose for which it was created, treating people as sexual objects, and emphasizing parts of the body over the person's intrinsic worth and value."[9]

Pornography is addictive. In her book *An Affair of the Mind,* Laurie Hall says, "Porn is more addictive than cocaine or alcohol. Porn sends its tentacles in deep. It wraps itself around a basic physical need (sex), entwines itself in a basic emotional need (to be in control) and enmeshes itself with a basic spiritual need (for intimacy)."[10] Dr. Harry Schaumburg, author of *False Intimacy: Understanding the Struggle of Sexual Addiction,* adds, "A sexually addicted person becomes fully absorbed with sex, for it becomes the greatest need—not the greatest desire. Sex is wanted, demanded, and will be pursued at any cost."[11]

Pornography is progressive. Most men initially engage in noninteractive pornography—magazines, videos, and viewing pictures over the Internet—and progress to interactive porn such as live viewing at arcades, strip joints, or lingerie-modeling studios. Soon, the thrill from these experiences is gone, and the user seeks sexual contact (affairs or prostitution). Serious abusers go one step further and commit violent crimes. A study at the University of California at Los Angeles found that 51 percent of male students exposed to violent pornography indicated a likelihood of raping a woman if they could get away with it.[12]

Pornography draws the viewer into a destructive world of fantasy. In a letter to us, dated 26 August 1997, Dr. James Dobson, former member of the Attorney General's Commission on Pornography and founder of Focus on the Family, said the fantasy associated with pornography can have serious negative consequences on a marriage. "The stimulation of reality loses its ability to compete with the excitement of fantasy and a couple's sexual relationship is damaged."

Laurie Hall describes what she witnessed firsthand in her home.

> Over a period of time, the lines between what is fantasy and what is real become so blurred that the one affected can actually slip into a form of insanity. His mind begins a process of dissolution as his thoughts track only one way. The unused part of the mind begins to wither and die, and he gradually loses his ability to think deeply about the issues of life. Eventually, he becomes an empty shell of a man. Hollow to the core, he wanders aimlessly through life, seeking only one thing: fulfillment of the lust that has taken complete hold of him.[13]

Pornography leads to death. "Pornography kills the soul, steals the heart, and destroys the mind."[14] Pornography puts to death marital intimacy and destroys families. Those who engage in prostitution or affairs expose themselves and their spouse to *physical death* through the possibility of contracting a deadly sexual disease. But all pornographic users face certain *soul death* because pornography severs fellowship with God and kills moral consciousness.

Pornography is a mistress, an adulteress. Her goal is to rape your husband's soul and lead him to the grave.

> For the lips of an adulteress drip honey, and her speech is smoother than oil; but in the end she is bitter as gall, sharp as a double-edged sword. *Her feet go down to death; her steps lead straight to the grave.* (Proverbs 5:3-5, NIV, emphasis ours)

Imagine for a moment that your husband is standing in front of a door that leads to the dungeon of death. Satan gives him a key labeled "pornography" and says, "Go to the dungeon. Exciting things are happening down there, things you don't want to miss." Your husband uses the key to unlock the door, then takes his first step down the dark, spiraling stairs. He watches a racy movie. Step two. He studies naked women on his computer monitor. Step three. He dials up phone sex. Step four. Down, down he descends, deeper into the inky blackness, farther away from you, farther away from God and those who love him. Closer to death. You stand at the top of the stairs calling his name. You want to help, but how? You can't go down after him. What can you do?

You can turn on a light.

TURN ON A LIGHT

Light is your only ray of hope to dispel the darkness. We are going to suggest you turn on six different lights. You will notice that these "lights" are directed toward you, not toward your husband. Why? Because the only person you can change is you. You can pray for your husband. You can encourage him to get help. But in the end, you cannot make decisions for him.

Our primary concern is to encourage you and to help you keep a "God-centered" perspective during this dark time. Ask God to speak to you as you read and to show you what is needed in your particular situation.

1. Turn on a light: Expose the enemy. In the darkness, it's difficult to tell who the enemy is. Is the enemy your husband? Is the enemy the naked blond beauty sprawled across the centerfold? Or the industry churning out the enticing images?

No. The real enemy is Satan. "For our struggle is not against flesh and blood, but . . . against the powers of this dark world and against the spiritual forces of evil in the heavenly realms" (Ephesians 6:12, NIV). Dr. Ron Miller reports in his book, *Personality Traits of the Carnal Mind,* "Willfully seeking after pornographic material opens up one's spirit to demonic influence and even control by an unclean spirit."[15]

Satan's nature is to lie, deceive, kill, and destroy (John 8:44, 1 Peter 5:8). He wants to kill your husband's spirit and destroy your family. He will try to deceive you into believing your husband is the enemy. Don't believe it! You and your husband need to stick together if you are going to win this thing. You CAN defeat Satan and win the battle against pornography if you continually rely upon God's strength. God specializes in changing people. He is more than capable of snatching His children from the claws of the enemy. "With God we will gain the victory, and he will trample down our enemies" (Psalm 60:12, NIV).

2. Turn on a light: Pray for your husband. Don't sit in fear, kneel in prayer. What should you pray?

In *Celebration of Discipline*, Richard Foster, author and professor of theology, says, "We can pray for sexual deviations with genuine assurance that a real and lasting change can occur. Sex is like a river—it is a good and wonderful blessing when kept within its proper channel. A river that overflows its banks is a dangerous thing, and so are perverted sex drives. What are the God-created banks for sex? One man with one woman in marriage for life. When praying for persons with sexual problems, it is a joy to picture a river that has overflowed its banks and invite the Lord to bring it back to its natural channel."[16]

Pray for God to bring your husband's sexual appetites back within the confines of the bank. Pray also for God to expose your husband's secret sins so that they may be found out. "There is nothing concealed that will not be disclosed, or hidden that will not be made known" (Luke 12:2, NIV).

SUGGESTED LETTER TO HUSBAND

My Dear Husband,

This letter is hard for me to write. I don't know exactly how to say what I need to, so bear with me! I love you. I am committed to you and to our marriage. I desire to be a creative lover. I want our sexual relationship to grow, but in order for it to grow, our lovemaking *has* to be just between the two of us. I believe that God created the sexual relationship to be enjoyed exclusively between a husband and wife, no one else. When another person is brought into our bedroom, whether that person is in the flesh, on a picture, in your mind, or in a video, our intimate encounter is no longer intimate. When we *(name the practice you object to)*, I feel violated and exposed. I pull away from you emotionally and physically, not because I WANT to, but because our intimate oneness has been destroyed. I want to love you creatively and freely, but to do so means eliminating *(name practice)* from our lovemaking. Thank you for respecting my wishes in this area. Again, I love you and am committed to growing in our love relationship.

Your wife

Pray, *God, you know what my husband does in secret and how secrets are harming our marriage. By the power of your Holy Spirit, please expose these sins so that he can get help.*

3. *Turn on a light: Read God's Word.* "The unfolding of your words gives light" (Psalm 119:130, NIV). One wife said, "In those dark days of dealing with my husband's pornography habit, the thing that comforted me most was reading God's Word."

Even though it may not feel like it, God is near and weeping with you. "The LORD is close to the brokenhearted" (Psalm 34:18, NIV). "God is our refuge and strength, an ever-present help in trouble" (Psalm 46:1, NIV). Take time to sit at His feet. If you can, take a whole day, go off by yourself, and pour your heart out to Him. Bask in the Psalms. Seek wisdom from Proverbs. Ask God to speak to you through His Word and to show you what to do (see Psalm 32:8, Proverbs 3:5-6).

4. *Turn on a light: Talk to a friend.* During a December 1997 interview, James Groesbeck, a licensed marriage-and-family therapist who has worked with those who have felt the pain of pornography, told us, "It is critical for a woman whose husband is involved with pornography to have a strong network where comfort is freely given and counsel is strong—including a discerning female confidante, a small group of trusted friends, and a competent therapist." You desperately need people who can emotionally support and advise you spiritually, relationally, and psychologically.

Groesbeck recommends intentional prayer and practical wisdom in choosing those who will be your "inner circle," as an unwise choice could make matters worse, resulting in poor counsel, unwelcome pain, betrayal, and broken confidences. "Hopefully," he adds, "a woman has already established such a network before she finds herself in crisis."

5. *Turn on a light: Clarify your boundaries.* We know several wives who have watched X-rated movies and gone to topless bars with their husbands because they didn't know how to set boundaries. In her book *The Christian Woman's Guide to Sexuality,* Debra Evans says, "You are not in ANY way obligated to act out sexual situations with your husband derived from a fantasy life fed by pornography. Period."[17]

Establishing boundaries is critical because, as Drs. Henry Cloud and John Townsend write in their book *Boundaries,* which we recommend:

"We need to keep things that will nurture us inside our fences (boundaries) and keep things that will harm us outside. . . . The concept of boundaries comes from the very nature of God" who defines what is good and what is not.[18] If you are unclear about God's boundaries concerning sexual practices, you will find help in chapter 17.

Let your husband know you want to be an exciting, creative lover for him, but that you are unwilling to cross certain lines, such as engaging in sex if he visits a strip joint. Another necessary boundary in today's disease infested society, is to protect yourself against sexually transmitted diseases. If he has been with another woman, you may need to cut off all sexual contact until he is remorseful and can prove he is medically safe.

6. Turn on a light: Examine your heart. "Search me, O God, and know my heart; try me and know my anxious thoughts; and see if there be any hurtful way in me, and lead me in the everlasting way" (Psalm 139:23-24). Examining yourself is often the most difficult part of helping your husband fight the battle of pornography. Examining yourself means prayerfully and honestly answering tough questions. For example:

- Do I have any behaviors or attitudes toward sex or my husband that have been harmful to our marriage relationship? Pray Job 34:32 (NIV): "Teach me what I cannot see; if I have done wrong, I will not do so again."
- Am I judging my husband or looking down on him for this sin? Consider Matthew 7:1 (NIV): "Do not judge, or you too will be judged."
- Am I withholding forgiveness? Matthew 6:14-15 (NIV) says, "For if you forgive men when they sin against you, your heavenly Father will also forgive you. But if you do not forgive men their sins, your Father will not forgive your sins."
- Am I so focused on my husband's addiction that I am failing to deal with my own addictions? Matthew 7:3-4 (NIV) says, "Why do you look at the speck of sawdust in your [husband's] eye and pay no attention to the plank in your own eye? How can you say to your [husband], 'Let me take the speck out of your eye,' when all the time there is a plank in your own eye?"

➻ Is God pleased with how I am handling this situation? Pray Psalm 19:14 (NIV): "May the words of my mouth and the meditation of my heart be pleasing in your sight, O LORD, my Rock and my Redeemer."

Remember, there is no condemnation for those in Christ Jesus. Trust God to lovingly correct and instruct you as you work through this situation.

LET THERE BE LIGHT!

> Who walks in darkness and has no light? Let him trust in the name of the LORD and rely upon his God. (Isaiah 50:10, NKJV)

> He reveals deep and hidden things; he knows what lies in darkness, and light dwells with him. (Daniel 2:22, NIV)

In the darkness, it's easy to doubt that God is at work. The Israelites did. Night hung over the Israelites like a heavy wool blanket. Their ears strained in the blackness, listening. On one side, thundering horse hooves reminded them that the Egyptians were nearly upon them. On the other side, the rhythmic lapping of the Red Sea seemed to whisper, "You're trapped . . . trapped." Mothers hugged children to their breasts. Men counted the minutes, knowing each could be their last. All pondered the inevitable—death or, at the very least, enslavement.

Meanwhile, God was at work. He moved the pillar of cloud from the front of the Israelites to the back so it came between the two armies. Tucked away in Exodus 14:20 (NIV) is the phrase, "the cloud brought darkness to the one side and light to the other side." Even though night had fallen, God supernaturally gave the Israelites light, allowing them to see the dry path on the floor of the sea. Hope dawned as they saw a way of escape.

Like the Israelites, do you feel trapped? Are you hugging your children to your breast, fearing the death of your marriage? Do a host of emotions pursue you, intent upon enslaving you? As surely as God was at work for the Israelites, He is working for you at this moment. Ask Him to continue His work in your heart, in your husband's heart, and in your marriage. "My God turns my darkness into light" (Psalm 18:28, NIV). Will you pray?

O God, You know my heart is breaking; every part of me is breaking. I know the answer is to turn to You and trust You, but I feel so weak. Give me the power through Your Spirit to trust You in this night of darkness. Be my refuge and strength, my present help in trouble. I need You so much.

CHANGE MY HEART, O GOD

1. Plan a "Day with God." Pack your Bible, a notebook, pen, and any other helpful resource material and go off by yourself to be with your Lord. During your time, memorize Psalm 32:8 (NIV): "I will instruct you and teach you in the way you should go; I will counsel you and watch over you."

2. While you are alone with the Lord, specifically ask Him to direct you to your pastor, a trusted friend, or counselor who will share your burden with you.

3. Review the six lights and ask God how you can apply these in your situation.

HOW CAN I KNOW IF MY HUSBAND IS
INTO PORNOGRAPHY?

Unlike a drug addict or an alcoholic, there are no needle marks or telltale breath to know if someone is addicted to pornography. How can you identify a pornography user?

Following are some behavior indicators that suggest possible involvement:

Emotional isolation. The compulsive viewer of pornography is physically and emotionally detached. Addicts can appear social and even "the life of the party," but they hold people at arm's length and avoid intimate relationships.

Lying. Addicts lie to cover up their habit. This practice often carries over to other areas of the user's life such as finances, accomplishments, and intentions.

Compulsive behavior. Users often exhibit extreme behaviors in other areas of their lives, such as compulsive buying, exercise, diet, or work.

Demanding, selfish attitude. Pornography is about lust, not love. The goal of the user is to satisfy himself and his needs. The more prolonged the exposure to pornography, the greater the selfishness on the part of the user.

Increased defensiveness and anger. Because many addicts are successful at hiding their "secret," they feel they don't have to be accountable to others about any behavior. Thus, when confronted with *any* issue, they respond with abnormal anger and defensiveness.

Lack of respect for women. Heavy users exhibit an increasing attitude of superiority over women and frequently treat them in a demeaning manner. Women become viewed as objects whose primary function is to serve the addict. Also, addicts tend to "undress" women with their eyes, indulging in long, lingering looks.[19]

Though a wife may find these behaviors extremely hurtful, the man addicted to pornography does not set out to intentionally hurt his spouse. His actions are often rooted in his own emotional pain. Dr. Harry Schaumburg, in his excellent book *False Intimacy: Understanding the Struggle of Sexual Addiction,* says, "It isn't just an issue of sex or even of external behavior: It's a byproduct of loneliness, pain, the self-centered demand to be loved and accepted regardless of the consequences, and a loss of vital relationship with God."[20] If you suspect your husband is into pornography, resist the temptation to snoop around for evidence. Such actions sabotage marital trust and violate privacy boundaries. We know it is scary, but trust God to bring what is hidden into the light. "There is nothing concealed that will not be disclosed, or hidden that will not be made known" (Luke 12:2, NIV). His timing and methods are best.

ROMANCE NOVELS: PASTIME OR PORNOGRAPHY?

Many excellent Christian romance novels are available on the market that are free of sexual innuendos and violence. However, not all romance novels can be classified as harmless reading material. The following is taken from a letter sent to *Focus on the Family* magazine:

> I hear so many warnings about pornographic magazines, pornography on the Internet, etc. But what about the so-called "romance novels"? These books are sexually explicit, they contain violence of a sexual nature, and they are also addictive. There was a time when I couldn't put them down. I had a tendency to shut out my family and ignore my responsibilities.
>
> I read this material for years before, and after, becoming a Christian. It caused problems in my relationships and my marriage. My husband hauled the novels out of our home by the boxful. . . . These books are not hidden behind counters. There is no age limit on their availability. Children can purchase them in the grocery store. Can you warn people, especially parents, of these books and the potential damage they can do?[21]

For recommended resources regarding pornography, see page 258.

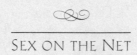

SEX ON THE NET

Pornographic material from the Internet comes to our homes in two ways: unsolicited and solicited.

Unsolicited material is dropped in your electronic mailbox from uninvited vendors the same way you receive junk mail. An estimated 30 percent of the 30 million daily unsolicited pieces of e-mail floating around is pornographic or racist.[22] The computer user must decide whether to respond to the mail or throw it away.

Solicited material is something the computer user seeks. A user might go to his "browser" or "find" command and type in "Playboy" or any other word that could route him to the more than 70,000 websites that offer pornographic material.

How can you protect your home from pornography?

Set ground rules in advance. Talk with your husband (and kids) and establish "Family Computer Rules" that spell out reasonable content and time restraints. A content restraint might be "We agree as a family to dispose immediately of pornographic junk mail and not to visit websites or chat rooms where the topic is sexual in nature." A time restraint might be "We agree not to use the computer after 10 P.M." (Isolation increases temptation, and statistics show increased pornographic activity late at night and early in the morning.)

Use screening devices. Screening devices come in several forms: software you can install in your computer that monitors computer activity or restricts access to certain areas, websites that monitor or restrict certain activities, and screening capabilities you may place on your computer's "browser." The combination of these three tools will make it more difficult to access pornographic material, but be aware that no method is 100 percent foolproof. There are ways around most locking devices, and software that blocks specific websites must be regularly updated because new sites are added to the Internet daily. For recommendations for the most up-to-date screening software, contact your local library, school, or computer store. The Center for Democracy and Technology has a website that provides information about blocking and screening programs. Its address is http://www.netparents.org.

Monitor activity. The filing cabinet in your e-mail program keeps a list of every e-mail received. The "bookmark" feature on your computer's browser shows which websites were last visited, and the history file on your computer's hard drive can tell what files have been accessed, by whom, and when.

Ultimately, whether your computer is used to access pornographic material is a matter of the integrity of the user. A wise wife does not make herself paranoid playing computer cop, but she discusses the dangers with her family and makes sure certain checks are in place.

fourteen

Is It Possible to Get Beyond the Pain of Sexual Abuse?

*I*f you have turned to this chapter because you have been a victim of sexual abuse, we want you to know something: *We've spent many hours praying for you.* The more we pray, the more we are convinced that your greatest need is not for *human wisdom,* but for *divine healing.* Because we desperately want to see you set free from the bondage of your past and to enjoy a healthy sexual relationship with your husband in the present, we feel the best thing we can do is to "get out of the way" and allow God's Spirit to speak directly to you. He knows your needs. He knows your wounds and how to heal them. We pray that each word written here will serve as a funnel through which God will pour forth His truth and love to you. Will you pray the following prayer?

> *God, You have heard my plea for help and have had me turn to this chapter for a reason. You know how I long to be free from my past, but no matter how hard I try to get over what has happened, the pain won't go away. Sometimes I hurt so much I think I will die. Other times I feel numb, as if I am already dead. I want to be healed, but I don't want to think about what's happened. Help, God! You are my only hope. You know how hard it is for me to trust anyone—even You. But where else can I go? You alone have the power to heal me. Speak to me as I read. Show me what to do. Give me hope that I truly can be free of this pain and enjoy sexual love with my husband in the way You intended it to be.*

HOPE FOR HEALING

Sadly, sexual abuse is becoming increasingly common in our society. Experts cannot agree on the actual number of victims, only that the number is high. Sarah, an accountant and mother of two was a victim at a young age. She told us:

> I was eight when my brother's friend, thirteen, raped me twice. One night at dinner I told my parents that this boy had pulled down his pants in front of me and they went crazy! They were so upset I knew I could never tell them what had *really* happened. I was so confused. Part of me actually liked some of the things I felt, but mostly I felt ashamed because I knew what had happened was wrong. In being raped, I lost more than my virginity; I lost my childhood. From that moment on, I felt different from other girls. I remember my friends giggling about sex and imagining what it must be like to kiss a boy. I knew so much more. Even at ten I could pick up sexual innuendos from guys that other girls had no clue about.
>
> My brother knew about the rape, but instead of defending me or avenging me, he teased me. I hated him for that. I found myself suspicious and distrustful of all men.

Sarah's story is heartbreaking, but not unusual. If you weren't sexually abused yourself, it's likely you know a woman who has been. Sexual abuse varies in type and intensity, but all sexual abuse results in a multitude of painful issues for the victim. We are unable to address all these issues in one chapter, so we have included a list of helpful resources on page 259. Instead, we will focus on one issue only, the single most important question you must answer: *Do you believe God can heal you of your sexual abuse and bring you into a satisfying, intimate relationship with your husband?*

Perhaps you want to believe God can heal you, but something is holding you back. Maybe you are like the man who took his son to Jesus to be healed. Jesus said, "Everything is possible for him who believes." The father's reply was: "I do believe; help me overcome my unbelief!" (Mark 9:23-24, NIV).

Dear friend, it is our hope that today you will overcome your unbelief. How is this possible? How do we move from unbelief to belief? It happens when we rid our mind of lies, replace the lies with God's truth, and entrust ourselves to the One who is trustworthy. Please understand. We are not attempting to oversimplify what can be a very complicated process. Complete healing often takes years and involves sorting out a tangled web of emotions and thoughts. But thousands of abuse victims will tell you *healing is possible!* And healing begins with trusting God.

THE GREATEST LIE

Perhaps you'd like to trust God, but because of the violation you have suffered, trust does not come easily. To make matters worse, Satan, the enemy of your soul, doesn't want you to trust because he doesn't want you to be healed. He fights to keep you in bondage to your pain and does everything in his power to keep you trapped by your past. Why? Because other wounded women might hear your testimony and turn to God.

Scripture warns us not to be ignorant of Satan's schemes, to stand firm against him, and to resist his lies (2 Corinthians 2:11; Ephesians 4:27; 6:11). Lies are Satan's most effective weapon. He lied to the first woman, Eve, telling her that she would not die if she ate of the forbidden fruit in the Garden of Eden, and he has been lying ever since. He lies to you. He lies to us. He lied to Sarah and tried to destroy her.

Sarah told us that in college she found herself becoming increasingly angry and moody. Something was going on inside of her, something evil, but she could not put her finger on it. She said: "I wanted so badly for someone to love me, but I knew no one ever would. I felt worthless. I cried all the time. I couldn't concentrate on my studies. I found myself slipping deeper and deeper into a black hole I couldn't crawl out of. Several times I tried to kill myself."

Sarah did not realize that she had an adversary who was intent on destroying her, telling her that no one would ever love her and that she was worthless. Satan would have been thrilled if Sarah had taken her life.

If you are a Christian you need to realize that, as with Sarah, Satan is intent on destroying you. The Bible tells us he is like a roaring lion who seeks to devour you (1 Peter 5:8). He continually accuses you (Revelation 12:10). He lies to you and about you because that is his nature. Listen to

Jesus' description of your enemy. "He was a murderer from the beginning, and does not stand in the truth, because there is no truth in him. Whenever he speaks a lie, he speaks from his own nature, for he is a liar, and the father of lies" (John 8:44).

Make no mistake, lies are Satan's favorite tool for keeping you in bondage. Each lie Satan gets you to believe becomes a link in a chain that he wraps around you. When you struggle to be free, Satan tugs on the chain. The links tighten, suffocating you with pain and fear. The length of the chain and the shape of the individual links are different for every victim of sexual abuse. But regardless of the length and strength of your chain, *Jesus can set you free.* He proclaims:

> The thief comes only to steal, and kill, and destroy; I came that [you] might have life, and might have it abundantly. (John 10:10)

> You shall know the truth, and the truth shall make you free. (John 8:32)

> I am the way, and the truth, and the life. (John 14:6)

Jesus is the *way* out of your pain. He is *truth.* When we exchange Satan's lies for His truth, the chains fall off and we have *life.*

Are you tired of feeling dead inside? Are you sick of your chains? Do you want to be free? Then don't dillydally. Let's look at a lie, the whopper of all lies—the lie Satan perceives to be the strongest link in his chain—get rid of it and replace it with the truth.

Lie:

Satan: "God doesn't care about sexual abuse, and He certainly doesn't care about you. Otherwise He would have intervened and stopped your abuser."

Truth:

Jesus: "God loves you. He hates sexual abuse and is deeply grieved over what your abuser did to you. God will punish your offender, and His punishment will be just. God earnestly desires to heal you and set you free."

THE GREATEST TRUTH

You are already familiar with Satan's lie, so let's not waste time dwelling on it. Instead, let's focus on God's truth and the four thoughts it contains.

1. God loves you. Think of the most pure, tender expression of love you have ever experienced and multiply it a thousand times. Even this cannot compare with the unconditional and limitless love God has for you. If you are a believer in Christ, you are God's precious child. Nothing you could ever do would make Him stop loving you. No place you could ever hide would put you outside the boundaries of His love. Dear precious child of God, let this sink into your soul and down to the tips of your toes. GOD LOVES YOU! We agree with the apostle Paul who says: "I pray that you . . . may . . . grasp how wide and long and high and deep is the love of Christ, and to know this love that surpasses knowledge" (Ephesians 3:17-19, NIV). Perhaps you don't *feel* God's love, but like the love of a mother who deeply loves her child even though the child may not feel it, love is there. Whom will you believe—Satan, who says God doesn't care about you, or God, who says, "I have loved you with an everlasting love" (Jeremiah 31:3)?

2. God hates sexual abuse. God created sexual love to be enjoyed between a husband and wife *only*. In the Old Testament, serious sexual crimes were punishable by death (Deuteronomy 22:22). God prohibited sex among family members. In fact, He said it was a sin to even *think* about such a thing. "No one is to *approach* any close relative to have sexual relations" (Leviticus 18:6, NIV, emphasis ours). "Everyone who does any of these detestable things—such persons must be cut off from their people" (Leviticus 18:29, NIV). Some offenders were literally "cut off," as in Deuteronomy 25:11-12 where a woman's hand was to be cut off if she seized the genitals of a man who was not her husband.

These verses show us that God established clear boundaries concerning sex and deadly consequences for those who violated them. Whether your abuser was a friend, a relative, a neighbor, or a stranger, God abhors what that person did to you. Perhaps you are thinking, *If God feels this strongly about sexual abuse, why didn't He stop my abuser?* We realize that there is no emotionally satisfying answer to this question, but there *is* an answer. God didn't stop your abuser because when He created us God gave us the gift of free will.

Your abuser chose to use this gift in an evil way. God is deeply grieved over your abuser's actions, but because He is true to His word, God will not take back a gift He has given. BUT, He will heal you (if you allow Him) and punish your abuser. Our society does not punish sexual offenders with the severe penalties God originally proclaimed. But though we fail to enact earthly punishment, God will not fail to bring about heavenly justice. "His works are perfect, and all his ways are just" (Deuteronomy 32:4, NIV).

3. *Your offender will be punished.* In fact, in God's eyes, your abuser has *already* been punished. In our humanness, we cannot comprehend a God who lives outside the boundaries of time. For God, past, present, and future are one. Your abuse, your anguish, your healing, your abuser's judgment are one complete picture in God's framework. Because you are stuck in time, you cannot see what God sees. You look at the brushstrokes around you, and they don't make sense. Even standing on your tiptoes and peering into the future as far as you can, you see no justice, so you conclude justice is not in the picture. This, however, is Satan's lie. What is God's truth?

> It is mine to avenge; I will repay. In due time their foot will slip; their day of disaster is near and their doom rushes upon them. (Deuteronomy 32:35, NIV)

> He repays a man for what he has done; he brings upon him what his conduct deserves. It is unthinkable that God would do wrong, that the Almighty would pervert justice. (Job 34:11-12, NIV)

> Be sure of this: The wicked will not go unpunished. (Proverbs 11:21, NIV)

> Vengeance is mine . . . saith the Lord. (Romans 12:19, KJV)

Beloved, be certain: The punishment your offender will suffer will be more severe than even you might expect because God's standards are much higher than our own. God may allow you to witness your offender's punishment in this lifetime, or He may not. Either way, know that one day we must each stand before the judgment seat, and what God proclaims will be just.

4. *God desires to heal you.* One of God's names in Hebrew is *Jehovah Rapha,* which means "the God who heals." God's nature is to heal, as can

be seen through the life of Christ who came to heal and to save. God wants to heal you, but healing requires that you reach out and touch Him and that you allow Him to touch you. "And all who *touched* him were healed" (Matthew 14:36, NIV, emphasis ours).

We are not referring to a physical touch but to a spiritual touch—a touch in the deepest part of your soul where your strongest passions and emotions lie. Because your abuser wounded you in this tender place, you have built up a protective wall around this area to keep others out. The wall has successfully kept out those who would hurt you, but it has also kept out God, who longs to heal you.

God is not like your abuser. He doesn't want something from you, He wants to give to you. He has gifts for you, gifts of joy and freedom, gifts of love, acceptance, and purpose. He wants to hold you and comfort you, but unlike your abuser, He will not touch you against your will. He will not force Himself upon you or demand that you love Him.

So, He waits. He waits for you to turn to Him, waits for you to extend your hand and receive the gifts He longs to give.

Oh friend, God's heart breaks over what your abuser did. But there is something that grieves Him even more, and it is this: *You are afraid to trust Him.* You do not love Him with all your heart, soul, mind, and strength. Your focus is upon your suffering and doing everything you can to keep from being hurt again rather than trusting the One who loves you and wants to heal you.

The choice is yours. If you choose to pour your emotions and energies into things other than God, God will respect your wishes. But if you choose Him, He wants nothing held back. Trust Him! He is trustworthy.

WHEN WE DECIDE TO TRUST GOD

Sarah wanted to trust God, but secretly doubted His ability to help her. After all, He hadn't helped her at the time of the rape, what could He do now, after the fact? A turning point came in college when several friends, concerned about the severity of her depression, suggested they get together and pray. Pray they did—for three and a half hours. During that time, God did much healing. Sarah describes what happened.

I had not connected my attempted suicide to the rape, but as my friends prayed for my depression to lift, I suddenly found myself transported back in time to the garage where the rape took place. I wept uncontrollably; I didn't want to be there, but God whispered, "Don't run away. Trust me." Then a strange thing happened. The rape was taking place in front of me, but it was as if it were happening to someone else, not me; I was a bystander. I saw the eight-year-old girl lying on the cement. The older boy was on top of her. A chain bound them together at their wrists. Hovering over their naked bodies were two black clouds, one cloud was filled with lust and the other with anger. Suddenly Jesus was there. He was mad! He ordered the clouds away. Then He reached for the chain that bound the boy and girl together and snapped it in two. With the clouds gone and the chain broken, all that remained were two innocent and frightened children.

Another sexual abuse victim, Paula, describes her decision to trust God as a tremendous "leap of faith."

I remember wanting to jump off the high diving board at our pool when I was a little girl, but I was terrified. I'd walk to the end of the board, look down at the water, and freeze. Often I chickened out and went back down the ladder. One day I decided I'd jump off no matter what. I did, and surprise! I didn't die. In fact, I remember getting out of the pool thinking, *Why was I so afraid?* Trusting God was like jumping off that board.

My father had sexually assaulted me when I was a teenager. *Father* was a bad word in my book, so how could I trust God, who called Himself "Father"? I struggled for years to resolve this mental conflict and never could. I knew the only way I'd ever trust God was to do what I did at the pool, close my eyes and jump in with both feet. I did. It was the best decision I ever made. God is not *anything* like my dad. My only regret is that I did not turn to Him sooner.

Sarah and Paula trusted God with their past. Neither was healed instantaneously, but for both, healing began with taking a giant step forward to trust God. Now they had to take another big step: to trust God to take sex, the source of pain in their past, and use it to bring joy in the present.

WILL SEX EVER BE WONDERFUL?

Dan Allender, sexual abuse counselor and author of *The Wounded Heart,* writes, "I have never worked with an abused man or woman who did not hate or mistrust the hunger for intimacy."[1]

Your hunger for intimacy should never be despised. It is a God-given passion, a desire He intended to be satisfied, in part, through loving sex with your husband. How can you get over your mistrust of this longing? For many victims, it happens once they are able to exchange the sordid sights and sounds connected with their abuse for lovely sights and sounds connected with their spouse. Paula and Sarah explain.

Paula: "My ability to enjoy sex depended upon the pictures I saw in my head. When the pictures were pleasant, sex was good. But when the pictures were disgusting, I couldn't stand for Steve (my husband) to touch me. I got to the point I didn't even want to have sex because I was afraid a memory would come that I couldn't handle. One day I read 2 Corinthians 5:17 (NKJV), 'If anyone is in Christ, he is a new creation; old things have passed away; behold, all things have become new.' I saw that the 'old things' weren't passing away because I had not allowed any 'new things' in. It was like I had a photo album filled with horrible pictures. Throwing out the bad pictures wasn't enough; I needed new pictures to put in their place. Steve and I read the Song of Solomon together, then memorized several verses. As we made love, we spoke the verses to each other and talked about the beautiful picture we were creating. It was so romantic! Ironic, isn't it? My abuse actually forced us into deeper intimacy because we had to work so hard at making each touch beautiful and meaningful."

Sarah: "What bothered me most about the rape were the sounds: the boy above me grunting; the sound of my shoes, which he hadn't bothered to take off, sliding on the cement; my brother's mocking laugh; the horrified gasps of my parents. Worst of all were the sounds in my head that screamed, *You are dirty, used. No one wants you.* I knew if I was ever to be healed, I had to silence the sounds. Several things helped. When my husband and I made love, we played soothing piano music in the background. And I memorized several scriptures like Colossians 3:12 so when I heard in my head, *You are worthless,* I could say, *I am not. I am holy and dearly loved by God.* Sex is still not perfect. Like all couples, I guess we have to work at it to make it what we want it to be. But my physical relationship with my husband is better than I ever dared to hope for, and with God's help I believe it will only continue to get better."

GOD'S HEALING WORD

Paula and Sarah both cite reading and memorizing God's Word as a means for promoting healing of their past. Other abuse victims affirm this practice. As one woman shared, "Thoughts connected with my abuse were disturbing and evil, but thoughts in God's Word were comforting and good." Many scriptures refer to God's ability to restore what man had stolen, to take wickedness and turn it into something good.

> You meant evil against me; but God meant it for good. (Genesis 50:20, NKJV)

> The God of all grace, who called you to his eternal glory in Christ, after you have suffered a little while, will himself restore you and make you strong. (1 Peter 5:10, NIV)

> I will repay you for the years the locusts have eaten. (Joel 2:25, NIV)

> I would have despaired unless I had believed that I would see the goodness of the LORD in the land of the living. (Psalm 27:13)

> "For I know the plans I have for you," declares the LORD, "plans to prosper you and not to harm you, plans to give you hope and a future." (Jeremiah 29:11, NIV)

HEALING IS FOR YOU

Over and over, God takes what humankind meant for evil and uses it for good. Time and again, He transforms unspeakable acts of wickedness into something glorious. What better example than the crucifixion and resurrection of His son?

Today God wants to crucify (put to death) your past and resurrect you to a new life. New life begins when you place your trust in God. Many issues are connected to your abuse, but you don't need to think about them right now. The only question that needs answering is this: *Do you believe God wants to heal you, and, if so, are you willing to let Him begin that process today?*

Dear sister in Christ, hold back no longer! Fall at His feet and release your despair to Him. Let go of the lies, the pain, the anger. Trust Him. It is our earnest prayer that in the future you will look back on today as the day you found hope, the day you trusted God. Won't you pray to Him now?

> *Dear God, today I give to You the pain of my past, the confusion in my present, the hopes of my future. All that I am, all that I have, all that I suffer, I offer to You.*

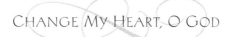

CHANGE MY HEART, O GOD

1. Select one of the hope-filled verses on page 172, and commit it to memory.

2. If you have never talked to anyone about what you have suffered, consider getting professional help. Ask your pastor for a referral, or contact one of the resources listed on page 259.

3. Remember that healing is a process and often involves hard work and intensive counseling. Don't give up when you encounter temporary setbacks. Meditate on 1 Timothy 4:15 (NIV): "Be diligent in these matters; give yourself wholly to them, so that everyone may see your progress."

∽

A FORMER MISS AMERICA ISSUES A WARNING

Marilyn Van Derbur Atler, Miss America 1958, was a victim of incest. Her mother was silent while her father abused her from ages four to eighteen. She cautions mothers: "We have to be willing to handle some stark truths. Our relatives are most often our violators. We teach our daughters to beware of the strange man in the park, but most children are sexually assaulted in the home or by someone who's trusted—a relative, a coach, a family friend."[2]

As mothers, we must educate our sons and daughters at an early age:

Explain the difference between appropriate touching and inappropriate touching. Many parents avoid discussing this because of embarrassment, but you cannot let uncomfortable feelings prevent you from this important discussion. Perhaps using a doll or teddy bear to explain the "off limits areas" would lessen the discomfort. Be sure to be specific and point to the genital area of the doll and name the parts that should not be touched. Then ask your children to tell you, using the doll and pointing to the body parts.

Tell our children they don't have to do anything that makes them feel uncomfortable. Sometimes Uncle John says, "Come give me a kiss." Or Grandpa urges your youngster, "Come sit on my lap." Certainly these can be appropriate actions, but Mrs. Van Derbur Atler says if we sense our children are uncomfortable giving this type of affection, we should not force them.[3]

Leave the door open for our children to talk with us. Make sure your child understands that if anyone—a baby-sitter, a teacher, a relative, another child, or adult—suggests inappropriate touching, you want them to say no and immediately come and tell you. Say to your child, "Honey, I love you. You can talk to me about anything. If anyone touches you inappropriately, I want to know because I want to protect you. I am always here for you."

You can never be too cautious when it comes to leaving your child alone with someone else. We have heard too many horror stories of parents who have left their children with caregivers they considered trustworthy and honorable, only to later discover their child had been sexually abused. The best protection you can give your children is to educate them and to allow honesty and openness about sexual issues to characterize your relationship.

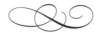

Sizzling Questions

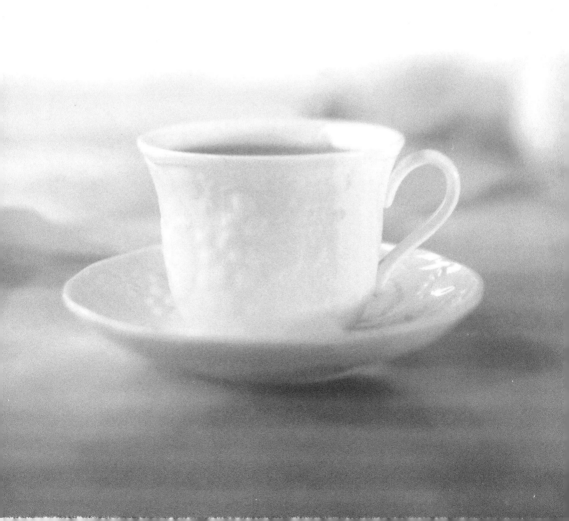

How Can Sex Go from Boring to Sizzling?

I (Linda) walked away from the Bible study feeling ridiculed and put down. I had been married five years and was teaching about the priorities of a woman's life. That morning I had made the statement that our relationship with our husbands should continue to grow in every area, including the sexual. An older woman laughed and condescendingly quipped, "Linda, you're young and naive. Just wait until you've been married twenty years. Sex gets old—you'll see."

I wish I could find that woman today. After thirty-five years of marriage, I'd like to look her in the eye and tell her that she was wrong. The sexual relationship can remain exciting. (Or, like she said, it can be boring. It depends on what we choose.)

In researching material for this book, we learned an interesting bit of trivia: Reportedly, a young woman yawned continuously for five weeks.[1] Five weeks without closing her mouth! This is quite a record, but many women we talk to indicate their sexual relationship is like one long yawn: BOR-ing!

Ho-hum sex would bore anyone. What is ho-hum sex?

- ❧ Always making love the same way. "I touch you, you touch me. Do this three times, then move on. Blah, blah, blah . . .
- ❧ Always making love at the same time—after the 10:00 P.M. news every Tuesday.
- ❧ Always making love in the same place—in bed, in the dark, and under the covers.

Do you feel a yawn coming on? Isn't the thought of doing the same thing over and over again, well, boring? Sadly, boredom reigns in many bedrooms. Does it in yours?

Anything can become boring. Think about it. If you are like every wife we know, you have probably gotten bored with cooking, cleaning, driving carpool—and sex. So what can we do? We each have a choice: to continue cooking plain spaghetti or to graduate to pasta Alfredo.

What's true in the kitchen is true in the bedroom. A wise woman told us, "If I was still cooking the same five meals I prepared when we were newly-weds, we'd dread eating. Over the years I've spiced up my recipes and added variety." Every "sexual meal" needs spice and variety. Are you still serving the same sexual meals you made your first year of marriage, or have you spiced up your menu?

The best way to put zip back into your lovemaking is to add a generous helping of creativity. But where do we go for our creative ideas? We know a book that is guaranteed to put the sizzle back into your sexual relationship. Its recipes for erotic, holy sex will stimulate your creativity and stir up your passion. The good news is, you probably already have several copies of this book in your home. If not, buy one immediately. In it you will find the most creative sexual advice given since the beginning of time. Ready for the name of the book? The Bible.

Before we show you some things you may have never before seen in your Bible, we need to get one thing straight—the Bible is the book we Christian women should turn to for all issues in our life, especially sex. The Author of the book created sex; He knows how our bodies and minds work. We need to quit listening to what the world says is sexy and romantic. Much of what is presented in magazines and on TV is immoral and a dark, fuzzy shadow of what God intended. So study His Book, your Bible.

GOD'S VIEW OF SEXUAL CREATIVITY

Walk with us through several scenes in the Song of Solomon as we look at God's view of sexual creativity. We think you will be amazed at the creative use of items like fragrance, poetic words, dance, and "dates."

1. Creative use of fragrance. At the beginning of the Song, Shulamith says, "Your oils have a pleasing fragrance, your name is like purified oil" (Song of Solomon 1:3). She describes her lover as being like the fragrant henna blossoms that grew in the oasis of Engedi (1:14). Obviously, the king used a tenth century B.C. version of Aramis or Brut.

Shulamith, too, was an expert in the application of perfumes. She says, "While the king was at his table, my perfume spread its fragrance" (1:12, NIV). She describes her hands as dripping with myrrh, then adds that Solomon was like the sachet of sweet-smelling myrrh that hung between her breasts (1:13, 5:5).

While their lovemaking creatively involved all five senses, it particularly emphasized scent. If we walked into their bedroom, we would immediately be greeted by the aroma of burning incense. The bedsheets, perhaps even the walls, would have been sprinkled with scented powders. Their bodies and their private place of lovemaking were especially prepared to give delight to the senses.

How can women today do this? Few couples in the twenty-first century sprinkle their walls with scented powders. I (Linda) am allergic to most fragrances and would make a quick exit from the bedroom if incense and powerful perfumes wafted from every corner. But all of us can find creative ways to enhance the atmosphere through the sense of fragrance. Here are just a few:

- Scented candles in French vanilla, spiced apple, wild berries, or evergreen mist. Myriad possibilities await you in every candle shop.
- Perfumes and colognes for her and him. Perhaps a fragrance used only during lovemaking—a special message to your husband that says, "My heart is set on loving you."
- Lotions of exotic aromas can be incorporated into lovemaking. An all-body massage with peppermint lotion appeals to our sense of smell and touch.
- Potpourri placed in the bedroom can create a fresh and vibrant fragrance.

2. Creative use of words. As the lovers inhaled sweet fragrances, they breathed out words that enveloped them in an aroma of love. Creative use of words set the mood for creative lovemaking.

Creative compliments. Solomon: "How beautiful you are, my darling! Oh, how beautiful! Your eyes are doves" (Song of Solomon 1:15, NIV). Shulamith: "How handsome you are, my lover! Oh, how charming!" (1:16, NIV). The lovers compliment each other with tender, warm words. As they explore each other's bodies, their words heat up. Solomon: "Like a lily among the thorns, so is my darling among the maidens" (2:2). Shulamith: "Like an apple tree among the trees of the forest, so is my beloved among the young men" (2:3).

The king praises his lover by picturing her as a supple, graceful lily, saying that all other women are like thorns compared to her. She responds by comparing Solomon to an apple tree, a symbol used in the Near East for sexual love. In essence, Shulamith is telling her husband what a skillful lover he is. Her words fill Solomon with an urgency to pleasure her sexually.

Now their words melt into steamy, passionate whispers. Solomon: "Your stature is like that of the palm, and your breasts like clusters of fruit. I said, 'I will climb the palm tree; I will take hold of its fruit.' May your breasts be like the clusters of the vine, the fragrance of your breath like apples, and your mouth like the best wine" (7:7-9, NIV). Shulamith: "Sustain me with raisin cakes, refresh me with apples, because I am lovesick. Let his left hand be under my head and his right hand embrace me" (2:5-6).

CAN AMERICAN WOMEN SIZZLE?

Has our culture taught us to be boring lovers? According to marriage counselor Mary Ann Mayo in *A Christian Guide to Sexual Counseling*, "The Chinese and Indians have always viewed the female as highly sexed and have trained them to be responsive and assertive partners. Western culture has portrayed the female as the passive sex partner. It is not surprising that American women believe and act as if they are not as captivated by sex as their men."[2]

How can American women change their mind-set from boring to sizzling? By continuing to seek God's perspective on sex, a perspective that does not change or vary from culture to culture. God urges, "Eat, friends; drink and imbibe deeply, O lovers" (Song of Solomon 5:1).

Shulamith is telling Solomon, "Here is how I want you to touch me." Many wives find it difficult to find the right words to say, "Love me like this." Shulamith communicated her sexual desires via poetry. When she said, "I am lovesick," she was literally saying, "I am sick with love, completely overcome with sexual desire." In order to alleviate the "lovesickness," she requests her husband to sustain her with raisin cakes and apples (symbols of erotic love). A modern counterpart might be, "Honey, I am ready for you. Come into me and satisfy me."

Shulamith then tells her husband exactly how he should satisfy her lovesickness, or sexual passion. She instructs him to place his left hand under her head and embrace or fondle her with his right hand.[3] Through the means of poetic expression, this creative wife tells her husband she desires him to fondle and stimulate her by touching her body.

Perhaps you are thinking, *My husband would laugh uncontrollably if I said, "Sustain me with raisin cakes!"* You're right. Our husbands would laugh too. But we should not dismiss the action because the words don't suit us. God saw fit to include these lovers' secret moments in His Word so we might have an example of how to use erotic and sensuous language appropriately in our lovemaking.

3. Creative names. Solomon and Shulamith devised poetic descriptions so they could communicate when it was hard to find the right word. Solomon's genitals are called fruit in Song of Solomon 2:3 and hers a garden in 4:12-16.[4] The poetic metaphors enabled the lovers to freely communicate in the midst of passion without feeling uncomfortable. When God spoke of personal aspects of sex, He could have used the slang terms, which raise a psychological censor in some, or medical terms, which leave a feeling of awkwardness and mechanics. The Lord avoided both problems by using poetic symbolism. This created a freedom of expression. Shulamith could speak to her lover of the "spices of her garden being wafted abroad." She could ask her husband "to eat of her garden's fruit."

Shulamith invites:

> Make my garden breathe out fragrance, let its spices be wafted abroad.
> May my beloved come into his garden and eat its choice fruits!

Solomon responds:

> I have come into my garden, my sister, my bride; I have gathered my
> myrrh along with my balsam. I have eaten my honeycomb and my
> honey; I have drunk my wine and my milk. (Song of Solomon
> 4:16–5:1)

How can you create private names so sexual communication with your
husband is more comfortable? Borrow garden and fruit from Solomon's
Song and make them yours. Or, discover your own personal names. Spend
time before making love devising special names that only you and your
beloved know. These secret names make it possible to communicate in the
bedroom and the kitchen, in private or in public. Instead of *garden*, one husband used the word *flower* to refer to his wife's vagina. She would call him
at work and say, "I have a bouquet of flowers for you tonight," or she would
hug him in the kitchen and say, "Honey, the flower is in bloom tonight."
(This husband worked overtime to get the kids bathed and in bed!)

The words you choose need to appeal to both you and your husband.
At first, you may feel awkward using your new names or phrases, but don't
give up. Couples who use their own private love language say that it not
only enhances their lovemaking, it makes them feel closer to each other
because they share an intimate secret no one else knows.

4. Creative use of dance. If you were startled by this biblical couple's creative use of names, get ready for another surprise. In chapter 6 we read that
Solomon and Shulamith are alone in the palace and Shulamith desires to
make love with her husband. As part of their love play, she aggressively
takes the initiative and arouses her husband's interest by provocatively
dancing before him. In a coy way she says:

> Why would you gaze on the Shulammite as on the dance of
> Mahanaim? (Song of Solomon 6:13, NIV)

Mahanaim was holy ground, the site where an angelic host appeared to
Jacob on his return to the Promised Land. Shulamith seems to be suggesting that her dance contained something as magnificent as an "angel" dancing before Solomon.[5] Certainly this angel was very seductive as Solomon
responds with these words:

> How beautiful are your feet in sandals, O prince's daughter! The curves
> of your hips are like jewels, the work of the hands of an artist. Your
> navel is like a round goblet which never lacks mixed wine. (7:1-2)

Commentators agree that "the curves of your hips" refer to their sway-
ing motion as she dances before Solomon. A modern day translation could
be "the vibration of the thighs."[6] The word navel is assuredly an incorrect
translation, probably reflecting the translator's modesty. The clear meaning
is that Solomon views his wife's garden (the poetic term for vulva) as she
dances nude—or in transparent garments—before him. Solomon says his
wife's garden never lacks mixed wine. Throughout the book, wine is used
as a symbol of sexual pleasure. It would appear that Solomon is suggesting
that her garden is a never-lacking source of sexual pleasure for him.[7]

Don't be embarrassed about the thought of dancing before your husband. Remember, it has God's stamp of approval. This is a description of
married love in the Bible. (Perhaps we should all run to Victoria's Secret
and buy a suitable "dancing outfit.") The message is clear. It is not only
acceptable in God's eyes for a wife to be aggressive sexually, and visually to
excite her husband, it is good. God designed the male mind (and other
parts of his body) to respond to visual images. Shulamith filled her husband's eyes with images that sent him into ecstasy. Are you ready to do the
same for your husband?

5. Creative use of dates. In these next verses, we see Shulamith planning
a weekend escape to the mountains of Lebanon with her beloved. There,
in the lovely springtime beauty she will give herself to him.

> Come, my beloved, let us go out into the country, let us spend the
> night in the villages. Let us rise early and go to the vineyards; let us see
> whether the vine has budded and its blossoms have opened, and
> whether the pomegranates have bloomed. There I will give you my
> love. The mandrakes have given forth fragrance; and over our doors
> are all choice fruits, *both new and old, which I have saved up for you,*
> *my beloved.* (7:11-13, emphasis ours)

It appears that this creative wife is inviting her husband to join her for
a time of lovemaking in the forest. She not only suggests they make love

outdoors, she entices her lover by saying the mandrakes (considered an aphrodisiac in the ancient world) are in bloom. "Oh, Solomon, the spring-time atmosphere of the countryside is conducive for lovemaking—be prepared for surprises, my love. Not only have I saved up sexual pleasures you are accustomed to, but new sexual pleasures also await you!"

What a creative wife. Shulamith skillfully built her husband's sense of anticipation by appealing to his sexual imagination. We're certain that this lucky husband replayed the countryside scene in his mind many times, wondering with excitement what the new pleasures would be.

What can we learn from this skillful wife?

Be aggressive in planning "sexual escapes" for you and your husband.

Be creative in communicating the surprise, thus building anticipation.

Be innovative in saving up new as well as old sexual pleasures for your lover.

CREATE THE NEW

What do you desire? You can stay in your BOR-ing, ho-hum mode, or you can enter into the fresh newness of creativity. It begins with the way you mentally see your sexual relationship. Stephen Covey, author of *The 7 Habits of Highly Successful People*, says that all things are created twice, first mentally and then physically. The key to creativity is to begin with the end in view, with a vision and a blueprint of the desired result.[8]

What result do you desire? Who do you want to become as a lover? Where do you want to be five years from now? Ten years?

It has been said that you can become a Rembrandt at your sexual art or you can stay in the paint-by-numbers stage. For some this is like leaving the city of our comfort and going into the wilderness. When Shulamith danced provocatively before Solomon, it must have been a "wilderness experience," and yet her creativity sparked excitement and enthusiasm in her husband and added flavor to their lovemaking.

Perhaps you have been waiting for the spark of creativity to just "happen" in your sexual relationship. Or maybe you are waiting for your husband to make it happen. If you wait, what will happen is BOR-ing. But if you make a decision to go forward, to introduce creative activity into your love life, the zip will come. Are you brave enough to live creatively in your sexuality? Like Shulamith, will you offer both "old and new" sexual delights to your husband? You can serve the same flat fare day after day, year after year, or you can create something new and exciting!

Dear Lord, I know our sexual relationship has been boring and I've done little to add creativity. Forgive me and give me the courage to step out and be creative. Show me specifically what I can do to add spice to our love life. I desire to be like the wife in the Song of Solomon. I can't do it alone, I desperately need Your help.

CHANGE MY HEART, O GOD

1. Do you creatively incorporate all five senses—touch, smell, taste, sight, hearing—in your lovemaking? Choose one sense you'd like to develop further and ask God to show how you might do this. (You will find some helpful examples on pages 229-30.)

2. Suggest to your husband that you read the Song of Solomon together and discuss ways you can grow in creativity as a couple.

3. Read again how Solomon and Shulamith creatively used fragrance, words, poetry, dance, and "dates." Commit to use creativity in one of these areas this week.

4. Invite your husband to an "Evening of Passion" with you. Build his sense of anticipation by providing him with a menu beforehand that includes the main course (you), a tantalizing dessert (something new), and entertainment (piano music, a Shulamith dance—use your imagination!). You might want to include that admission is free and clothing is optional.

What's the Big Deal About Orgasm?

A recent magazine trumpeted the following message across its cover:

MULTIPLE ORGASMS

COME-AGAIN GUIDE TO HELP YOU CLIMAX OVER AND OVER

READ THIS, GRAB HIM, AND HEAD TO BED

Another magazine related the humorous story of a couple enjoying their first vacation in a charming inn without the baby. The new parents felt sex-deprived and let things get a little out of hand. Anne relates:

> In my ecstasy, I kicked the antique crystal lamp on the bedside table, HARD. It went flying, taking along the vase of hydrangeas next to it. Both hit the floor with a resounding crash. Moments later, the owner of the inn appeared at the door with her cleaning cart. The next morning, a humiliating note at the front desk asked us to vacate the premises as this was a "wholesome family business" and we were not the desired clientele.[1]

Kicking a lamp over because the orgasm is so intense, climaxing over and over—it sounds like a fantasy—and for many women, it is. According to a 1994 Sex in America survey conducted by the National Opinion Research Center at the University of Chicago, nearly one-quarter of American women never achieve orgasm and another half only climax occasionally. This means almost three-quarters, or more than fifty million of us, go without orgasm either some or all the time.[2]

When climaxing is difficult, the last thing we want is a magazine blaring at us about "mutliples." We don't want to hear about shattered lamps when it takes all our energy just to experience a mild current of electricity. With the media shouting about orgasms and millions of women struggling in this area, it's no wonder the experts report that orgasm anxiety is one of the top sexual concerns among women.[3]

Maybe you've never had an orgasm, or maybe orgasm is difficult for you. In this chapter, we want to explain what orgasm is, how it works, and suggest some things you can do to move your body toward orgasm. But first, it is important that we have a proper perspective about the subject.

MAKE "SOULGASM" YOUR GOAL

We have said throughout this book that there are two perspectives on sex— the world's view and God's view—and that these two views are often diametrically opposed. Generally speaking, the world sees orgasm as the goal of lovemaking. In the past twenty-five years, orgasm has become the hot topic. Women have been encouraged to come out from under their Victorian covers and experience the "Big O." Hundreds of books and articles have been written about how to make orgasm happen. In the early 1950s, Alfred Kinsey (of the "Kinsey Report on Sexuality") helped people understand the physical aspects of orgasm. In the 1970s, Masters and Johnson built upon this physical dimension and added a clinical emphasis. Certainly some of what these experts have said has been helpful, but in the imparting of information something was left out.

Dr. Paul Pearsall, author of *Super Marital Sex,* believed that what had been omitted was the emotional element. He suggested the word *orgasm* be thrown out because it had come to mean only a physical response. He coined a new word, *psychasm,* in an attempt to merge the physical and emotional aspects. He said, "Sexual intercourse and all sexual interaction is one of merging rather than penetration."[4]

Dr. Pearsall was on the right track when he married the physical and emotional aspects of orgasm, but even he left something out—the spiritual. Orgasm is a powerful force, uniting a man and woman at the deepest levels of physical, emotional, and spiritual intimacy. We'd like to coin our own word to describe this wondrous union—*soulgasm*. Soulgasm is the sexual enjoyment between a husband and wife in which the physical, emotional, and spiritual intertwine and fuse the couple into soul oneness. This oneness is so complete that, in the eyes of God, the man and woman are no longer two distinct persons, but one being (Genesis 2:24).

The world sees orgasm—and the physical release that accompanies it—as the goal of lovemaking. But God sees the goal of lovemaking as something much more grand. Lovemaking is not just a series of ecstatic sensations, but truly loving one another.

Scripture does not talk about the physical release that takes place during lovemaking. It does, however, talk about the intimate emotional and spiritual oneness with a spouse—soulgasm (see Ephesians 5:31). Theologian and Christian sex therapist, Dr. Douglas Rosenau, says it well, "The purpose is not having intercourse or achieving an orgasm. The purpose of the lovemaking process is to unite with your one-flesh companion as God designed—with anticipation, warmth, excitement, mutual pleasure, and intimate bonding."[5]

We are not in any way diminishing the importance of the physical aspect of orgasm. In fact, we have devoted much of this chapter to a discussion of the physical orgasm and how we can encourage our bodies to give in to it. Rather, we want to elevate the importance of the emotional and spiritual so that all three carry equal weight. Orgasm is the frosting on the cake, not the main ingredient. Still, because the frosting is so tasty, it bears further investigation.

What Is Orgasm?

The root meaning of the word *orgasm* means to swell or be excited. Webster defines orgasm as "the ultimate emotional and physical excitement of a sexual act."

Dr. Rosenau says an orgasm is "a reflexive response; it is not an intentional act of your will. You cannot consciously will yourself to have an orgasm. Orgasms are a product of sufficient buildup of physical, mental, and emotional stimulation as the mind focuses on that increasing sexual tension."[6]

Wives who have experienced orgasm offer their less clinical definitions:

> "Waves of pleasure flow over me; it feels like sliding down a mountain waterfall."

> "Orgasm is the most tension releasing time of my life. Stress evaporates. A rush of pleasure engulfs me. I feel totally relaxed, at peace, and in love."

> "It's like having a million tiny pleasure balloons explode inside me all at once. The pleasure explosion continues for about twenty seconds, then calms, leaving my body tingling from head to toe. When the tingling stops, I sigh. I wish the feeling could go on forever."

Orgasm is wonderful, but it is only one element of lovemaking. Sex researchers Masters and Johnson identify orgasm as one of the four phases of the lovemaking cycle. A four-phase cycle can sound like the engineering lingo for combustion but actually it is the exciting process our bodies move through during the lovemaking process. Let's look at each phase.

1. Excitement. The initial stages of arousal are called excitement. For the man, this is displayed through a swelling penis; for a woman it is a moist vagina (this varies with women and during the aging process; some women do not experience moistness). During this phase, a woman's nipples become erect and her breasts swell. The outer third of the vagina becomes more engorged with blood, and the clitoris enlarges to two or three times its relaxed size.

2. Plateau. The second phase, plateau, is a bit of a misnomer because instead of excitement leveling off, it builds. For many couples this phase, which tends to be more spouse-centered, is often the longest and most enjoyable. The husband concentrates on pleasuring his wife, and she reciprocates. Back and forth they ignite the flames of passion in each other's bodies. Stephanie says, "My favorite part of sex is not the orgasm, but the pleasurable feelings that lead up to it. The building of sexual tension, then resting, then building again is filled with such intimacy and fun. The heights of orgasm are great, but if I had to name a favorite phase of lovemaking it would be the ever-growing sensations of passion before the release."

3. Orgasm. In the third phase, muscle spasms create heightened pleasure. While the husband is aware of his orgasm approaching, some women are not aware of when they will climax. As the husband and wife approach orgasm, each must concentrate on his or her own seuxal feelings. Orgasm is a reflexive action, and a woman must focus on her body and the building tension in order for her to climax. Suddenly, there is an explosive release in which muscles contract, creating beautiful sensuous sensations.

4. Resolution. After orgasm, tensions release, muscles relax, and the body returns to its original state before sexual arousal. There is great fulfillment in this phase as husband and wife learn to enjoy the pleasures of an extended resolution phase. One woman describes the joy of just relaxing together. "I think my favorite part of lovemaking is the 'afterglow.' We are sated with pleasure, limp and relaxed. My husband lays in my arms across my breasts and I massage his head or I lay across his chest and he softly caresses me. Sometimes we talk intimately, sharing the wonder of closeness and thanking our lover for the pleasure. Other times, we are quiet together. It is all beautiful."

Perhaps you are one of the women who have longed to experience all four stages but feel you've never progressed past phase two. For you, orgasm is an illusive dream hidden in your body and you want to find it. We'd like to suggest a few ideas that might help. Let's look at one of the most effective ways to increase orgasmic response.

EXERCISE YOUR LOVE MUSCLE

Your PC muscle (pubococcygeal) is your love muscle. Some women have never heard about this intriguing muscle. Others say, "I know all about the PC muscle." Maybe you learned about the PC muscle in childbirth classes but then forgot about it. But let us ask you—have you ever tried to strengthen it through exercises?

Let us give you a good reason to start a PC muscle exercise program. The PC muscle, or the "orgasm muscle," controls the intensity—and frequency—of your climaxes.[7]

Beverly Whipple, Ph.D., president-elect of the American Association of Sex Educators, Counselors, and Therapists, explains why a powerful PC muscle increases the likelihood of orgasm and makes your orgasms more intense. "The pubococcygeal muscle is like any other muscle. The stronger it is, the stronger the response—in this case, orgasm."[8]

One reason PC exercises increase your possibility of achieving orgasm is that when you exercise it, you mimic the natural muscle contractions that take place during orgasm. And the great thing about this exercise is that no jogging suit is required! You can exercise your love muscle without anyone knowing, sitting at your desk, standing at the sink peeling carrots, or relaxing in the bathtub.

How do you exercise the "orgasm muscle?" The next time you go to the bathroom, squeeze the PC muscle and stop the flow of urine. This is the muscle you will contract in your exercises. To strengthen the PC muscle, tighten it for three seconds, then release for three seconds. Do ten repetitions, three times each day. Work up to five-second holds three times a day. "Ultimately you should aim to do three sets of fifty contractions five to six days a week. When the muscle is in shape, you can cut your workouts down to three a week."[9]

Strengthening the "orgasm muscle" is not the only way to increase orgasmic response. Read on to discover six more secrets.

Six Secrets of Highly Orgasmic Wives

Different techniques work for different women. Try these suggestions and discover what works for you.

1. Grab your Nikes. In a study conducted by sex therapist, Dr. Linda DeVillers, 27 percent of women reported an increase in their ability to climax after beginning an exercise program. When the body is aerobically fit, the cardiovascular system works far more efficiently, producing increased blood flow to the genital area which can make orgasm much more intense."[10] The goal is not to scale Mount Everest, but to engage in twenty minutes of power walking or stationary cycling—or some other aerobic exercise—three times a week.

While exercise helps some women, the opposite approach helps others. "When my husband approaches me for sex and I'm bone weary, I suggest we sit in the bathtub together first and relax," shares Madeline, a wife of twenty-five years. "Soaking in the tub, sipping raspberry tea, and talking quietly with my husband erases my tiredness. When I'm able to relax first, I'm able to climax later."

2. Open your mouth. For the first three years of marriage, Mona "faked it." Finally, she got up her nerve and told her husband that while she enjoyed the warmth of lovemaking, she'd never had an orgasm—and she wanted to learn. Together they read books, prayed, and went on a treasure hunt of discovery. Mona learned the importance of honest communication with the man she loved.

One of the secrets of orgasmic wives is their ability to use the "C" word—communication. "The ability to tell her husband what feels good is directly linked to the likelihood of an orgasm. Women who are emotionally open have tremendous freedom to experience orgasm."[11] As one wife expressed, "I'm not afraid to tell my husband exactly what feels good because I know he wants to please me. I'm not just physically naked in the bedroom but emotionally naked too."

You are unique; your body is unique. This is why you must communicate what feels good to you. Take hold of your husband's hand. Show him where to touch you and how much pressure to apply. Let him know if you like circular rubbing, up and down stroking, or featherlike tickles.

3. Let yourself feel. In order to experience a physical orgasm, we must concentrate on pleasure, on the buildup of tension, and the increase in desire. As Christians, we often think that focusing on ourselves is wrong, that we should concentrate on giving, not receiving. But in order to move toward physical orgasm, we must give ourselves permission to dwell on our physical responses and emotional feelings. One woman told us, "We are suppose to be making love, but instead of focusing on my husband, if I want to climax, I have to focus on me. This makes me feel selfish."

But it is not selfish. Dr. Rosenau says great sex, like a good marriage, allows an individual to strategically focus on personal pleasure as well as the mate's. There is a fascinating paradox as your selfish inward journey to orgasm and intense personal excitement become a mutual experience and a marvelous turnon for your mate.[12]

4. Reduce genital paranoia. God says we are fearfully and wonderfully made (Psalm 139:14). The intricacy of God's design of the female body, including the genitalia is amazing. Yet women rarely speak the words "vagina" or "vulva," and many refer to their genital area as "down there" or avoid naming it at all. By contrast the Chinese use beautiful names; the vagina is the Jade Gate and the clitoris the Pearl of the Jade Gate.[13] We think adopting the Chinese words would help us see our genitals as also wonderfully made. A second benefit of these lovely phrases would be to promote communication during lovemaking. "Honey, touch my pearl and make my Jade Gate ready" is just easier to say than "Honey, touch my clitoris and make my vagina ready."

5. Be thankful. Melinda had never been able to experience an orgasm. She felt like her body was sexually dead, and she didn't know how to resurrect it. Melinda was discouraged, so was her husband. Instead of grumbling about never being able to achieve orgasm, she decided to try thanking God for every little thing. "If it felt good when my husband rubbed my cheek, I thanked God. If I liked it when he kissed me, I thanked God. When he touched my breast and I felt a teeny tiny sensation, I thanked God. It was wonderful because it changed my attitude about our lovemaking. It was no longer a time of 'Will I feel something?' but 'There *will* be something to thank God for.' Slowly, I began to tune in to my sexual feelings. It was a long process but I have now experienced orgasm. I believe thanking God had a lot to do with it."

6. Educate yourself. In an age where we are bombarded with sexual innuendos, we still miss understanding how the body works. We recommend two excellent Christian books that provide detailed information on orgasm for women. Ed and Gaye Wheat in *Intended for Pleasure* suggest the husband and wife enter an intimate training program together and work toward the wife becoming orgasmic.[14] In *A Celebration of Sex,* Rosenau includes three specific plans couples can work through to help the wife become more easily orgasmic.[15]

WHEN NOTHING WORKS

Maybe you've tried all these secrets and still have never experienced an orgasm. Should you give up hope?

Maggie had been to Christian counselors, desperate for help with her lack of sexual response. She'd exercised her body and PC muscle, read books, prayed, but she had never been able to have an orgasm.

When Maggie was fourteen, her promiscuous sister had died of AIDS. Full of grief and anger, Maggie's mother begged her never to be intimate with a boy before marriage. Wanting to honor her mother, Maggie stuffed all sexual stirrings deep inside her. When she married a wonderful man, she tried to reconnect with her sexual feelings, but they seemed lost forever.

Maggie came to me (Linda) in tears. "My husband Jim wants a responsive wife, but I feel nothing. I lie there like a board. I want to experience orgasm, but I can't begin to imagine what that would feel like. I feel like a failure."

I wept with Maggie over her heartache. Then I said, "I don't know why God has not answered and given you and Jim the joy of sharing the beauty of orgasm together. I trust that God knows best, but I don't always understand Him. You ask me what you can do. Maggie, orgasm is important but sex is more than explosive feelings of release. It is an intimate joining of body, soul, and spirit. Even if God never grants your request for physical orgasm, you can become a godly and sensuous lover to Jim. You can enjoy the giving and receiving of emotional pleasure. You can become an expert at pleasuring your husband. You can become his 'Shulamith.'"

Dear friend, wherever you are today, orgasms—experiencing "multiples" or struggling to experience one—should not be the sole focus of your lovemaking. The goal of lovemaking is not orgasm, but soulgasm, the fusing of you and your husband into a profound and beautiful soul-oneness. Every woman can experience soulgasm. Will you allow God to show you how?

Change My Heart, O God

1. Write in your own words a description of the word *soulgasm*.

2. If appropriate, ask your husband to read this chapter and discuss what it means to you individually and together.

3. Consider starting a PC muscle exercise program this week.

4. Pick one of the six secrets from highly orgasmic women that you want to apply this week.

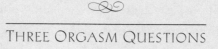

THREE ORGASM QUESTIONS

Is it true that orgasm is centered in the clitoris?

The Latin word for clitoris is "little key." For the majority of women, stimulation of the clitoris is the key to experiencing orgasm. Most doctors and experts agree with this, but some women have told us that for them orgasm is centered as much in the vagina as in the clitoris. Each woman is unique in the way her body responds.

Can women have multiple orgasms?

Yes. A woman may experience separate orgasms minutes apart, or during an intense lovemaking session with increasing arousal, she may experience them in rapid succession. This rapid succession can also be explained as a more intense orgasm, which can have ten to twelve spasms. Some women discover that as they reach the time of peak sexual expression for a woman (her late thirties), she is surprised by a second orgasm. This is what happened to Bethany:

> It had never occurred to me that I could come more than once. Then I read that this sometimes happened to women as they grew in giving in to their sexuality and in their trust of their husband. I think reading about it opened the door—and the next time we were making love I experienced wave upon wave of pleasure. As he entered me, I built up to another orgasm. It wasn't something I tried to make happen, but it was glorious, and my husband felt like "Superman lover."

How important is it to reach orgasm simultaneously with your spouse?

Some suggest that the epitome of lovemaking is to experience orgasm simultaneously. This is very difficult to accomplish as an orgasm is a reflexive response, not an intentional act of the will. You cannot say, "In three minutes we will both reach orgasm. Ready, set, go. One, two, three, BANG." One woman described trying to experience orgasm together as the same as trying to sneeze together—not likely to happen.

There is no "right way" to make love. The important issue is what is pleasurable to you and your husband. Some couples find that intercourse is more pleasurable for the women if she has already reached a climax as her genitals are lubricated and engorged. Each couple must discover the patterns that fit them best, individually and together.

seventeen

What's Not Okay in Bed?

The responses we received to our survey regarding the questions Christian women have about the sexual relationship in marriage ranged from "If both partners agree, is anything taboo?" to "What about the use of vibrators?" More than any other question, women asked, "Is oral sex okay?" But at the heart of each of these questions were two concerns: What does God prohibit in the sexual relationship between a husband and wife, and what does God permit?

As we mentioned in the introduction, in preparation to write this book we read the Bible from Genesis to Revelation and compiled a list of every scriptural reference to sex. As we reviewed our list it became apparent that God gives tremendous sexual freedom within the marriage relationship. But God also sets forth some prohibitions that we must honor.

GOD'S TEN PROHIBITIONS

These are the ten things God forbids:

1. Fornication: Fornication is immoral sex. It comes from the Greek word *porneia* which means "unclean." This broad term includes sexual intercourse outside of marriage (1 Corinthians 7:2, 1 Thessalonians 4:3), sleeping with your stepmother (1 Corinthians 5:1), sex with a prostitute (1 Corinthians 6:13,15-16), and adultery (Matthew 5:32).

2. Adultery: Adultery, or sex with someone who is not your spouse, is a sin and was punishable in the Old Testament by death (Leviticus 20:10). In the New Testament, Jesus expanded adultery to mean not just physical acts, but emotional acts in the mind and heart (Matthew 5:28).

3. Homosexuality: The Bible is very clear that for a man to have sex with a man or a woman to have sex with a woman is detestable to God (Leviticus 18:22; 20:13; Romans 1:27; 1 Corinthians 6:9).

4. Impurity: There are several Greek words which are translated as "impurity." To become "impure" (in Greek, *molvno*) can mean to lose one's virginity (Revelation 14:4),[1] or to become defiled, due to living out a secular and essentially pagan lifestyle (1 Corinthians 6:9, 2 Corinthians 7:1). The Greek word *rupos* often refers to moral uncleanness in general (Revelation 22:11).

5. Orgies: For a married couple to become involved in sex orgies with different couples is an obvious violation of (1), (2), and (4) and needs no discussion.

6. Prostitution: Prostitution, which is paying for sex, is morally wrong and condemned throughout Scripture (Leviticus 19:29, Deuteronomy 23:17, Proverbs 7:4-27).

7. Lustful passions: First, let us tell you what this does not mean. Lustful passion does not refer to the powerful, God-given sexual desire a husband and wife have for one another. Instead, it refers to an unrestrained, indiscriminate sexual desire for men or women other than the person's marriage partner (Mark 7:21-22, Ephesians 4:19).

8. Sodomy: In the Old Testament, *sodomy* refers to men lying with men.[2] The English word means "Unnatural sexual intercourse, especially of one man with another or of a human being with an animal."[3] Unfortunately, some Christian teachers have erroneously equated sodomy with oral sex. In the Bible, sodomites refer to male homosexuals,[4] or temple prostitutes (both male and female).[5] In contemporary usage, the term *sodomy* is sometimes used to describe anal intercourse between a man and woman. This is not the meaning of the biblical word.

9. Obscenity and coarse jokes: In Ephesians 4:29, Paul says, "Let no unwholesome word proceed from your mouth." The Greek word for *unwholesome* is very descriptive and literally means "rotten" or "decaying." In Ephesians 5:4, the Bible warns us to avoid "silly talk" or, as it is called in some versions, "coarse jesting." We have all been around people who can see a sexual connotation in some innocent phrase and then begin to snicker or laugh. This is wrong. However, this does not rule out appropriate sexual humor in the privacy of marriage, but rather inappropriate sexual comments in a public setting.

10. Incest: Incest, or sex with family members or relatives, is specifically forbidden in Scripture (Leviticus 18:7-18; 20:11-21).

Now that you've read the list, we are certain all your questions have been answered, right? Not likely! God leaves much in our sexual relationship with our husbands up to our discretion. In all likelihood, the questions tugging at the back of your mind were not even touched upon. When she read this list, Shelby commented: "It's helpful to know what God says is wrong, but I still sometimes wonder if what my husband and I are doing is right. We have a great time together in bed, but every now and then, this nagging doubt comes—does God approve?"

To help you and all the Shelbys, we will get more specific and address the questions we are constantly asked.

IS ORAL SEX PERMISSIBLE?

Clifford and Joyce Penner, in their excellent book *The Gift of Sex,* give this definition of oral sex: "Oral sex or oral stimulation is the stimulation of your partner's genitals with your mouth, lips, and tongue. The man may stimulate the woman's clitoris and the opening of the vagina with his tongue, or the woman may pleasure the man's penis with her mouth."[6] This sexual stimulation may or may not lead to orgasm for the husband and wife.

What does Scripture say about this sexual activity? Most theologians say the Scriptures are silent about oral-genital sex. Some believe two verses in the Song of Solomon may contain veiled references to oral sex. The first is Song of Solomon 2:3:

> Like an apple tree among the trees of the forest, so is my beloved among the young men. In his shade I took great delight and sat down, and his fruit was sweet to my taste.

Throughout the Song of Solomon, the word *fruit* refers to the male genitals. In extra-biblical literature, fruit is sometimes equated with the male genitals or with semen, so it is possible that here we have a faint and delicate reference to an oral genital caress.[7]

The second possible veiled reference is found in 4:16 (KJV):

> Awake, O north wind; and come, thou south; blow upon my garden, that the spices thereof may flow out. Let my beloved come into his garden, and eat his pleasant fruits.

These erotic words spoken by Solomon's bride are at the culmination of a very sensuous love scene. Shulamith asks her husband to blow on her garden (a poetic reference used throughout the Song for the vagina) and cause its spices to flow out. Of course one cannot be certain, but it is possible Shulamith is inviting her husband to excite her by caressing her with his mouth. She then invites him to enter her and feast on the pleasures waiting in her "garden."

Dr. Douglas Rosenau believes Scripture is silent on the topic of oral sex. "This does not make it right or wrong," he says.[8] A key emphasis in the New Testament is Christian liberty. Nothing is unclean in itself, says Paul (Romans 14:14), and this presumably includes sexual variety. Lewis Smedes, professor of theology at Fuller Seminary, amplifies Paul's statement about nothing being unclean.

> Christian liberty sets us free from culturally invented "moral" taboos; and since there is no rule from heaven, it is likely that the only restraint is the feeling of the other person. For example, if one partner has guilt feelings about oral sex play, the Christian response of the other will be to honor the partner until they adjust their feelings. On the other hand, if the partner has only aesthetic reservations, and if these are rooted in some fixed idea that sex is little more than a necessary evil anyway, they have an obligation to be taught, tenderly and lovingly, of the joys of sex in the freedom of Christ.[9]

In *Intended for Pleasure,* Dr. and Mrs. Ed Wheat say that oral sex is a matter that concerns only the husband and wife involved. If both find it enjoyable and pleasant, then it may properly fit into the couple's lovemaking practices. One goal of lovemaking is to fill a treasure trove of memories with delightful love experiences that will quicken your responses during your future times together.[10]

One minister's wife blushes happily as she recalls a memo her husband sent requesting her presence for an urgent "appointment."

> RUN DON'T WALK! YOU WON'T WANT TO MISS THIS EXCITING, DYNAMIC, GRIPPING, SLEEP-DEFYING MEETING. Details follow: Would you like to have a meeting in the bathtub? (Loving massage and oral sex included.)
>
> I love you,
> Your husband

One woman might feel horrified by the above playful interchange between a husband and wife. To her, oral sex is repulsive. Another may think the minister and his wife have a gloriously free, creative, and fun sexual relationship. She sees that oral sex adds a beautiful dimension to this couple's lovemaking.

Before we go any further, let us clarify our intent in this chapter. Are we suggesting you incorporate oral sex into your love play? No. *We are not making recommendations.* Instead, our purpose is to set out for you what Scripture prohibits and to encourage you to seek God's wisdom concerning His personal recommendations for your marriage.

Each couple is different. Each husband and wife unique. Because Scripture is either silent—or veiled—concerning this practice, the only way to discover what God allows for you is for you to ask Him. If you've never talked to God about your sexual relationship, now is a good time to start. You will not shock God. Remember, sex was His idea. God is a God of wisdom (Daniel 2:20). He promises that when we lack wisdom, if we ask Him, He will give it to us (James 1:5).

As you seek God's wisdom, you might find it helpful to ask these three questions about any sexual practice you and your husband are considering:

↝ *Is it prohibited in Scripture?* If not, we may assume it is permitted. "Everything is permissible for me." (1 Corinthians 6:12, NIV)

    ➤ *Is it beneficial?* Does the practice in any way harm the husband or wife or hinder the sexual relationship? If so, it should be rejected. "Everything is permissible for me—but not everything is beneficial." (1 Corinthians 6:12, NIV)

    ➤ *Does it involve anyone else?* Sexual activity is sanctioned by God for husband and wife only. If a sexual practice involves someone else or becomes public, it is wrong based on Hebrews 13:4, which warns us to keep the marriage bed undefiled.

Let's see how these questions can help when it comes to making decisions about certain sexual practices that are not specifically spelled out in Scripture.

ARE VIBRATORS PERMISSIBLE?

Some couples enjoy incorporating the use of sexual aids such as vibrators into their lovemaking. To find out if the use of a vibrator is right or wrong, let's apply the three questions. Is the use of a vibrator prohibited by Scripture? Is a vibrator beneficial to lovemaking? Does the use of a vibrator involve anyone else?

As we look at the list of ten prohibitions, we see that there is no scriptural reference that would prohibit the use of a vibrator. So if a vibrator enhances a couple's lovemaking and is used exclusively for the couple's private enjoyment, then it is permitted. Does this mean we are suggesting you run out and buy a vibrator? No. Again, *we are not recommending any sexual practice.* We are only trying to help you discern what is best in your marriage as you seek the wisdom of God.

WHAT ABOUT X-RATED VIDEOS?

Obviously videos did not exist during biblical times, so we will not find "Thou shalt not watch X-rated videos" in the Scriptures. (The same is true for vibrators.) But as we read through the list of the ten prohibitions, a red flag is raised. In number two on the list, *adultery* is defined as "looking on a woman to lust" whether the woman (or man) is on a video, in a picture, or in the living flesh. Secondly, number four on the list describes *impurity* as "moral uncleanness." X-rated would qualify as "morally unclean," thereby making them something God would disdain.

Now, let's apply the questions:

Are X-rated videos prohibited in Scripture? Yes, based on (2) and (4).

Are X-rated videos beneficial? Anything that promotes "moral uncleanness" is not beneficial.

Do X-rated videos involve someone else? Yes. You bring the man or woman on the video into your lovemaking.

Based on these answers, we could conclude that God wants us to stay away from X-rated videos.

We have considered three "gray areas," oral sex, vibrators, and X-rated videos. There are many others. We encourage you and your husband to prayerfully seek God's wisdom, study the list of ten prohibitions, and use the three questions to help you discern what to do in your specific situation.

As Christians we are simultaneously free and responsible. We are responsible to seek the best of the one we love, to think more highly of him and his desires than our own (Philippians 2:3-4). But we are also free to explore new territories of sexual delight.

WOULD YOU BELIEVE . . .

As is often the case, humankind's laws are often quite different from God's laws. Here are some of our lawmakers' prohibitions:

- Oral sex between a husband and wife is illegal in twenty-three states.
- In Hastings, Nebraska, it is against the law for couples to sleep together naked in hotels.
- In Bozeman, Montana, a law prohibits couples, if nude, from engaging in any sexual activity in their front yards after sundown.
- In Alexandria, Minnesota, it's against the law for a man to make love to his wife if his breath reeks of garlic, onions, or sardines.
- One lawyer in Georgia said, "About the only thing that is legal in Georgia is sex between married couples in the missionary position. And then it has to be behind closed doors."[11]

According to Dr. Lewis Smedes, "The Christian word on trying out a sexual practice that is not prohibited in Scripture is 'Try it. If you like it, it is morally good for you. And it may well be that in providing new delight to each other, you will be adventuring into deeper experiences of love.'"[12]

God has given you great freedom in your sexual relationship with your husband. Remember His words to Solomon and Shulamith: "Eat, friends; drink and imbibe deeply, O lovers" (Song of Solomon 5:1).

CHANGE MY HEART, O GOD

1. If your husband is agreeable, read this chapter with him (otherwise, do this on your own). Discuss any sexual practice you are currently engaged in or considering that causes either of you to feel hesitant. Then:

    ☞ Read through the ten prohibitions. Do any apply to your situation?

    ☞ Ask the three questions. Do these clarify a course of action?

2. Honestly answer the following questions:

    ☞ Am I permitting something in my sexual relationship that God prohibits?

    ☞ Am I prohibiting sexual practices God permits? (Remember God gives individual wisdom in this area.)

3. Are you troubled about something in your sexual relationship with your husband? James 1:5 (NIV) says, "If any of you lacks wisdom, he should ask God, who gives generously to all without finding fault, and it will be given to him." God understands your concerns. He wants to give you wisdom. Won't you take some time right now to talk to Him about it? (If the sexual issue causing you concern involves pornography—pictures, videos, or any other form—see chapter 13, "My Husband's into Pornography—What Should I Do?" You might find the suggested letter to a husband on page 154 helpful.)

Are Quickies Okay with God?
(and Other What-Is-Normal Questions)

*M*any women we talk with want to be reassured that their sex life is normal, which raises the question: What is a "normal" sex life?

In this chapter we want to look at four questions regarding a sexual relationship.

How often is enough?

Is intercourse the only "proper" way to have sex?

Is it okay to schedule sex?

Are quickies okay with God?

HOW OFTEN IS ENOUGH?

Americans value being "normal." Many people look to surveys to tell them how they are doing. Dr. Ed Wheat asked five thousand couples how often they had sex during a week. The average was two or three times per week.[1] Another survey revealed that 33 percent of one hundred married couples were having intercourse two to three times a month or less. In a 1989 survey by the National Opinion Research Center at the University of Chicago, married people under forty reported having sex an average of only six and one half times per month. Respondents of all ages had sex an average of four and three quarters times a month,[2] far less than the two to three times per week reported by Wheat.

We learned from reading the surveys that the highly educated have sex less often, and those who work sixty or more hours a week are about 10 percent more sexually active than those working shorter hours.[3] People living in Northeastern parts of the U.S. have less intercourse than in any other region of the country. Those living in the Northwest have the most.[4]

If we took all surveys as gospel truth, we'd be sure we were workaholics, not too educated, and lived in Boise, Idaho. Perhaps "How often is normal?" is not the right question. Perhaps a better question is, "What is a successful sexual encounter for you and your husband?" Success is what pleases you and your husband and meets your needs. Yes, the "average" American makes love 2.2 times per week, but the issue is not how often but how fulfilling.

In *A Christian Guide to Sexual Counseling*, Mary Ann Mayo says:

> Without question, it is more accurate to speak of successful experiences than normal ones. Performance has little to do with being successful. One wonders, then, why there are so many authors, experts, and personalities all extolling the virtues of multi-orgasmic marathons. . . . High performance may be a virtue for race cars, but it is not the essential ingredient in a successful sexual relationship.[5]

What, then, is "successful sex"? We like this definition: It is free, mature, creative, and integrated.[6] What do these words mean? We define them like this:

> Free—to give and receive sexual joy as God intended.

> Mature—wrapped in agape love that thinks first of one's partner and longs to give pleasure to the one loved.

> Creative—not bound by tradition or preconceived ideas but open to new vistas of expressing love.

> Integrated—the sexual life is the frosting on the cake of the total love relationship. It is interwoven into the fabric of the life of the couple.

As one wife explained: "Sometimes lovemaking is giving a good backrub or giving my husband pleasure and a sexual release even though I'm too tired to respond sexually (my husband calls this 'mercy sex')." At other times, lovemaking is wild, abandoned sex and explosive orgasms. Usually lovemaking means intercourse, but sometimes it means giving pleasure in other ways. A beautiful sexual encounter may look one way on Tuesday and very different on Friday. Successful sex really depends on what is pleasurable to both spouses.

Now let's tackle the second question dealing with different ways to experience sexual release.

Is Intercourse the Only "Proper" Way to Have Sex?

Mandy came to me (Linda) and said, "I've had surgery and Tom feels like he's on a sexual starvation diet. He's walking around like a time bomb with his testosterone ready to explode. But my doctor says no sex for three more weeks. Tom's ready to call 911—what do I do?" "Mandy," I said, "There are other ways to satisfy one another." She looked at me incredulously. "Really?" Then she blushed, and a look of guilt crossed her face.

There are many times during a couple's years of marriage when intercourse just isn't a possibility: after birth, following a disabling accident or surgery, during a serious illness to name just a few. Is a couple to abstain from all sexual expression during these times? Or what if a couple is just interested in variety and wants to love one another in ways that don't include intercourse? Is intercourse the only "real thing"? Is any other type of sexual release second-class?

In *A Christian Woman's Guide to Sexuality*, Debra Evans, an expert in reproductive health and family wellness, says that our bodies are designed to achieve orgasm without engaging in sexual intercourse. The Bible clearly promotes the value of regular sexual release (1 Corinthians 7:1-5), so it is important to examine the role pleasurable touch plays in satisfying a couple's sexual needs.[7]

Intercourse is just one of many forms of human sexual experience, yet many Christian married couples have a lurking suspicion that eye-to-eye intercourse is the only "proper" activity for Christian married people. Couples may discard inhibitions in the throes of passion, but the light of morning finds some of them wondering if they were just a bit unnatural the night before[8]—"I blushed when I remembered what we had done last night. What would my mother think—what would our pastor think— what did I think?"

If it is true that intercourse is only one of many ways to have sex, why do some couples feel guilty the morning after loving and satisfying one another in ways that exclude intercourse? Perhaps it is because well-meaning Christian authorities have taught that to express sexuality in ways other than conventional sexual intercourse is wrong.

Mary Ann Mayo says this attitude conflicts with God's depiction of the sexual relationship in the Song of Solomon:

> Well-meaning Christian authorities teach that to express sexuality in any way other than through conventional sexual intercourse is wrong. This conflicts with God's depiction of the sexual relationship in the Song of Songs. Nor does it make sense. To imply that the mouth, the tongue, or the hands were not made for sexual purposes denies creativity and the fact that people use body parts for a multitude of purposes. Jesus made it clear that it is not what goes into a man that matters, but what comes out. If this truth is extended to sexual matters, it seems to suggest that sin is more a matter of internal heart and soul condition than of body parts and their use.[9]

Of course this does not give permission to engage in sexual acts that are specifically forbidden in Scripture. (See chapter 17.)

The apostle Paul declared "that everything as it is in itself is holy. We, of course, by the way we treat it or talk about it, can contaminate it" (Romans 14:14, Message). As we guard our minds against contamination and set our hearts on holiness, God grants us enormous liberty. "It is for freedom that Christ has set us free" (Galatians 5:1, NIV). In Christ, we are free from sexual practices that enslave us and free for sexual enjoyment with our spouse. We are free to enjoy sexual variety. If intercourse is right and good in the marriage bed, why not a variety of other sexual play?

Sex is a form of play. Lewis Smedes, professor of theology at Fuller Seminary, says:

God made us body-people. Bodies are meant to play and—we can add—to be played with. There is nothing more natural than body play, and it would be strange indeed if body play were off-limits only for sexual activities. Christian liberty sets us free from culturally invented moral taboos and since there is no rule from heaven, it is likely the only restraint is the feeling of the other person.[10]

So to answer the question, intercourse is not the *only* "proper" way to have sex.

The third question deals with scheduling sexual encounters.

IS IT OKAY TO SCHEDULE SEX?

Recently I (Linda) was waiting for my suitcases to arrive at the airport. A young couple beside me were greeting each other, passion oozing out of every pore. Their touching was sensual, their looks electric. They were literally "making love" by the baggage carousel. I turned my eyes away but found myself drawn again to the young lovers. This is the way it's supposed to be, or so the movies say. Instant passion. Spontaneity.

Before a couple marries, they schedule dates, time to spend together. Depending on the circumstances, dates sometimes just "happened," but most of the time they were penciled on a calendar. Not only did we look forward to the fun activities, long talks, and walks, but we also anticipated the physical contact. One woman said, "I could only see my fiancé on the weekends, and all week long I replayed each hug, the moments his arms embraced me, and dreamed of being there again." Was it unromantic for this woman to "plan" time with her beloved? Of course not. Their crazy schedules demanded it. Why then, when we marry, do we think it is unromantic to schedule sexual encounters? Is it because it isn't like the movies where couples are seized with passion just by the sight of one another?

Do you think you and your husband should just gaze into each other's eyes at the dinner table and be swept away with passion? This scenario might happen when you are away for the weekend alone or out to dinner alone, but in real married life there are children seated around the table who seize you to help with their homework. There are dirty dishes to wash, phone calls to make, meetings to attend, and bills to be paid. Or after a heavy day of responsibilities, the only thing that seizes you is the desire for sleep!

For most married couples, spontaneous sex just doesn't happen. What is the solution? To make time. And making time means planning—yes, planning.

Instead of thinking, "How unspontaneous! How unromantic!" Consider having an attitude which responds, "How wonderful to care so much that we make the time!"

Sex therapist Dr. Janet Wolfe addresses the need to plan for sex:

> If sex with your partner happens spontaneously, fine. But usually in the course of a busy life it doesn't. Simultaneous arousal is almost as unlikely as simultaneous orgasm. Anything worth doing is worth scheduling—especially things that require some time and space and freedom from distraction. We schedule activities all the time, from tennis games and plays to grease jobs on our cars. Surely sex is just as important to our physical and mental well-being—not to mention our relationship!—as these other activities.[11]

Planning time for lovemaking doesn't mean forcing sex to happen but creating the opportunity for it to happen. When we plan sex, we are saying that sex is as important as watching football, going to the gym, and being with friends. Let's look at how planning time worked for two wives.

Janine said: "Putting a red circle around every Friday was like an aphrodisiac. By noon my mind had slipped into 'sexual gear' as I thought, *Today's the day; I can't wait until tonight.* I even began to do things I hadn't done in years—sending a racy e-mail to Peter's office or calling to let him know tonight was on my mind. I feared scheduling sex would be a boring drag. Instead, creativity and anticipation surprised me."

Anna adds fun and excitement to her sexual relationship by making appointments with her husband. Her definition of an appointment? "A special time set aside to love each other and have a long-drawn-out intimate oneness lovemaking session." Perhaps Anna and Nick will schedule an appointment for Friday night or Wednesday lunch or December 10 at 6:30 A.M. Days before they will remind each other of their engagement.

Reminders are private, but also public. Anna and Nick work in the same office, and Anna has been known to announce in front of coworkers, "Nick, don't forget our important meeting Wednesday at noon!" On the morning of the appointment, Anna presses her body close to Nick's, kisses him, and whispers in his ear that she is looking forward to their rendezvous at noon! By lunchtime they are excited and very anxious for their appointment.

Anna said scheduling sexual rendezvous together makes them feel like newlyweds. Anna and Nick are in their sixties. They have been married over forty years. Like Anna and Janine, we must

- take the time if it's available
- make the time if there is no time
- plan the time

We have seen that scheduling time for sexual encounters can actually improve a couple's sexual relationship. But the question remains, are quick sexual experiences acceptable for Christian couples?

ARE QUICKIES OKAY WITH GOD?

Women love romance, candles, and long, slow times of lovemaking. Men like that too. But men also love the intense delight of spontaneous sex without all the romantic ritual. Does this indicate a lack of love or caring? No. Listen to one husband's words:

> I love to jump in the shower with my wife and feel the pounding water hitting our bodies as we mesh together. Within minutes we're on the bathroom rug—it is such pure, raw delight. It makes me love my wife so much and feel so close to her.

One marriage counselor puts it like this, "There is a certain kind of spontaneity, surrender, and passion that men experience when they allow themselves just to have sex with their wives. This is often lost in a more conscious, slow, step-by-step lovemaking process. Men actually crave this lustful surrender as much as women crave the safety and tenderness of lovemaking."[12]

This quick version of lovemaking doesn't appeal to some women. Others love it. Some Christian women feel somehow it must be wrong. Can a few minutes of bodies coming together be an expression of love? It depends on your attitude. Much love and caring can be communicated in a few minutes.

Let's consider three very different ways to make love: hors d'oeuvre sex, home-cooked sex, and gourmet sex.

Hors d'oeuvre sex. This is the quickie we've just been discussing. Dr. John Gray, in *Mars and Venus in the Bedroom,* says, "While many books talk about taking time for the woman to have a pleasurable experience, none seem to talk about the man's legitimate need to not take a lot of time. To be patient and regularly take the time a woman needs in sex, a man needs to enjoy an occasional quickie."[13] By "quickie," we are talking about the act of sex taking around three to five minutes. Yes, it's quick, but like an hors d'oeuvre of potato skins or fried zucchini, it satisfies and whets the appetite for a good, regular meal.

Home-cooked sex. Hors d'oeuvre sex is nice once in a while, but the staple of most couple's sexual diet is home-cooked sex. Fifteen minutes to a half-hour of warmth, foreplay, and intercourse. John Gray says this type of sexual encounter takes thirty minutes to build to orgasm: five minutes for him, twenty for her, and then, five minutes more to enjoy the afterglow of lying together in love.[14]

Gourmet sex. This is the kind of sexual encounter women dream about. Long, lazy, luxurious romance with no responsibility except loving. This is what we wish we could have continually, but in real life it just isn't realistic. Two hours to make love doesn't usually happen on a Wednesday night after the kids are in bed. You're too tired, the day has been too long, and so you opt for hors-d'oeuvre or home-cooked sex. Yet gourmet sex is vital to the life of a marriage. These special encounters light a spark that carries a couple over until the next time. Gourmet sex rarely happens spontaneously but with planning it can happen.

Here are two suggestions. (1) Alternate the planning of your sessions of delightful gourmet sex. One month the husband plans a sensational evening, the next month the wife. You may decide this is so much fun that you'll take turns every two weeks! (2) We hear continually from women,

"I'm just not creative. I don't know what to plan." To help, we have included a suggestion—an Intimate Secret—at the end of this book. Our hope is that this will spark your own creativity and that you will plan times to feast together at a gourmet banquet of lovemaking.

Hors d'oeuvre sex, home-cooked sex, and gourmet sex. Three different types of sexual expression that comprise a couple's sexual recipe file. But how do you communicate to your mate which variety of sexual encounter you're in the mood for tonight?

Some couples simply say, "Let's have a quickie." Others have devised phrases that are their private love language but communicate clearly whether they are talking about hors d'oeuvre, home-cooked, or gourmet sex. One couple's code phrase for sex was "sailing." If the wife wanted to make love, she might say, "It's a sunny day. Would you like to go sailing?" Sailing was their way to say, "Let's have home-cooked sex." When one of them wanted a quickie, they would suggest a "speedboat ride." When a luxurious time of gourmet sex was desired, "How about going for a long cruise?"[15] Maybe you want to adopt this couple's creative communication style. Or spend an evening with your husband brainstorming ideas and come up with your own private love language.

GOD'S GIFT OF PLEASURE

Sex is God's gift to married couples. He desires that you experience a free, joyous, and growing sexual relationship with your husband, that your lover "be exhilarated always with [your] love" (Proverbs 5:19). Are we recommending you do the things discussed in this chapter? No. Only you and your husband can decide what is right for you. Our hope is to encourage you in the freedom that is displayed in the Song of Solomon, that you would truly feast on your love, and "Drink and imbibe deeply, O lovers" (Song of Solomon 5:1).

The questions we have addressed in this chapter—How often is enough? Is intercourse the only "proper" way to have sex? Is it okay to schedule sex? Are quickies okay with God?—are not specifically answered in Scripture. Some women would feel better if God had written, "Thou shalt have sex three times every week" and "Thou shalt schedule sexual encounters." It would be nice if God directly spoke to every situation we encountered, but as we stated in the previous chapter, when the Scripture does not directly speak, we must look at the overall perspective on sexuality expressed in God's Word. God gave the gift of sex for procreation, intimate oneness, knowledge, comfort, to guard against temptation, and for pleasure (see chapter 1). God said more about pleasure than all the other reasons put together. So when deciding what is "normal" for you and your beloved, ask, "What is pleasurable for us?" "What creates a successful sexual experience for us?"

Here is how one woman described her physical relationship with her husband:

> The word I think of when I picture our sexual life is "flowing." There is such a freedom with one another. No modesty. No barriers. Just a desire to give pleasure to the other. Sometimes our lovemaking will last hours, other times minutes. But it is all beautiful. Sometimes we schedule sex, sometimes it happens spontaneously. Usually we culminate our love in the act of intercourse, but sometimes we satisfy each other in other ways. It all feels right, like I said our love just flows. Our commitment to Christ is the center of our relationship. Sex certainly isn't the most important aspect of our marriage, but it adds a fire that glows in us from one encounter until the next.

This is what normal sexual pleasure looks like in this marriage. It may look very different for another couple.

What does sexual freedom look like for you? Will you pray?

> *Lord, keep me growing as a godly and sensuous woman. Keep me from worrying about what is normal and let me dwell on what is a successful sexual encounter for me and my husband. Give me knowledge and wisdom about what a free and joyous sexual relationship looks like for us.*

CHANGE MY HEART, O GOD

If your husband is willing, ask him to read this chapter, and then discuss the following questions together. If possible, do this exercise when you have plenty of time and are alone. If your husband does not desire to participate, answer the questions yourself.

- Am I satisfied with the frequency of our sexual encounters?
- Am I comfortable with giving and receiving orgasm in ways other than intercourse?
- How do I feel about scheduling sexual encounters?
- What place do hors d'oeuvre sex, home-cooked sex, and gourmet sex have in our sexual relationship? How do we communicate the type of encounter we desire?
- What does a successful sexual encounter look like for us?

⨯

nineteen

How Can I Recapture the Passion?

I yearn for a lover who will make my heart pound a mile a minute. My husband used to—but the thrill is gone. Things are quiet, calm, and—I might as well say it—dull as dishwater."[1]

Perhaps you can identify with this woman's yearning for renewed passion. You've been married five, ten, twenty years, or more. The movies paint a picture of couples with glazed eyes, locked in steamy embraces. Novels portray the heroine unable to control herself as pulsating passion sweeps over her. You wonder what's wrong with you. The tantalizing, heart-pounding passion is a memory. And you'd like it back!

So you pick up a magazine with quick-fix ideas:

- ⚓ Make love on top of the washing machine—during the spin cycle.
- ⚓ Paint your bedroom purple—the "passion color."
- ⚓ Make love on skis! (We read of one couple who did this. Do you think they got cold?)

Can these quick fixes help? They might ignite a spark (and we'll give you a few "sparks" at the end of this chapter). But we want you to consider more than sparks; we want you to consider fanning the flame of passion, a lifelong flame that will warm your marriage and keep the fire burning.

Passion is the fuel. But we need to think of passion in a different way than the movies and novels portray it. To do this, we must seek the true source of passion.

PASSION DEFINED

Webster's dictionary defines passion as "A compelling, intense feeling or emotion; love, ardent affection, amorous desire."

We see passion aplenty in the Song of Solomon. Intense feelings live on every page. God waits until the end of the book to reveal the definition—and the source of passionate love. He says passion is intense, it is invaluable, and the flame of the Lord is its source. Read the beautiful poetic definition of love and passion spoken by the bride, Shulamith, to her beloved.

> Set me as a seal upon your heart, as a seal upon your arm; for love is strong as death, *passion* fierce as the grave. Its flashes are flashes of fire, a raging flame [the very flame of the Lord]. Many waters cannot quench love, neither can floods drown it. If one offered for love all the wealth of his house, it would be utterly scorned. (8:6-7, NRSV, emphasis ours)

To help you grasp the beautiful depth of these verses, we've paraphrased them as follows:

> O my Beloved. Press me close to your heart. Wrap me in your arms and hold me tight as your most precious possession. Your love, strong as death, seizes me with an irresistible force. I give myself to this love and yearn to be wholly and completely absorbed by it. My love for you is violent, vigorous, unceasing. I could no more give you up than the grave would give up the dead. My passionate love is a flame not kindled by man but by the Holy God. It is a waterproof torch, a flame of fire that mighty waters cannot quench.

This passionate love described by Shulamith is rooted in the zealous love the Lord God Almighty has for us.

The same Hebrew word translated in Song of Solomon 8:6-7 as "passion" is often used in the Old Testament to describe the passion of God. Sometimes the word is translated as passion, other times as jealousy or zeal. Several times we find the phrase, "The zeal of the LORD" (2 Kings 19:31; Isaiah 9:7; 37:32). God's zeal, His passionate and jealous love for His people, is an all-consuming passion that is both intense and invaluable.

I have loved you with an everlasting love; therefore I have drawn you with lovingkindness. Again I will build you, and you shall be rebuilt. (Jeremiah 31:3-4)

God's love is intense, it is invaluable, and it continues to build us up. It always seeks, always pursues, always builds. Shulamith's earthly, passionate love for Solomon possesses the same fiery intensity of devotion as God's love.

Our friend, this is true passion. This is holy passion. An inexhaustible flame ignited by our loving God that always seeks the lover, pursues her, and builds the love. This passion begins in the inner core of the relationship and penetrates into every facet of our being until the fire of love burns brightly.

How do we ignite this flame of passion in our marriages? We begin by making passion a priority.

MAKE PASSION A PRIORITY

Dr. Paul Pearsall, author of *Super Marital Sex,* says:

> The marriage comes first. All other people and events come after the marriage. Children, parents, work, and play all benefit most by marital priority instead of marital sacrifice, because the marriage is the central unit to all other processes. If it is true that we reap what we sow, then marriages are in big trouble. . . . If we put as much time in our working as we allow for our loving, we would end up unemployed or bankrupt.[2]

Couples are searching for intimacy in their love relationships, but the harvest is meager for lack of planting and nurturing. Goethe was correct when he said, "Things which matter most must never be at the mercy of things which matter least."

We have both made a commitment to God's priorities for our lives; God first, our husbands second. That commitment includes our sexual passion with our husbands. We have vowed to become more exciting lovers to our husbands every year. Having the right priority—that our husband is number one of all the people on earth—is the foundation.

What is your attitude toward your husband? Is he a high priority? Do you see him as your lover or merely the children's father, the one who takes out the garbage and snores? Do you look at him with "lover's eyes" or with eyes that have seen him too many times and no longer really see? Has the intensity of commitment waned? Do you still seek him first, or is he the last thing on your heart and mind? Do you pursue him and work to build up the passionate love between you, or has your love life become a flatline?

Recapturing passion has first to do with your attitude about being a lover to your husband. Passion begins with priorities, not genitals. When was the last time you "interrupted" your husband's morning shower by saying, "In case I haven't told you lately, you are the most important person in my life." And then proceeded to give him pleasure?

Perhaps you're thinking, *Linda, Lorraine, what planet do you live on? No one can keep looking at her husband with "lover's eyes" in the midst of daily life. Are you saying, "Fling him on the floor in the middle of paying bills" or "Seduce him as you boil the macaroni"?* We agree that it's difficult to keep the passion burning, but not impossible. Sex isn't an event. It is an environment. We must make passion a priority and then set an atmosphere where passion can reign.

SET AN ATMOSPHERE FOR PASSION

Webster defines *atmosphere* as a "good feeling that the mind receives from a place." What feeling does your lover receive when he walks into your bedroom? Passion or panic? Desire or disaster? Too many master bedrooms look like the family garbage dump. The trashman doesn't come on Tuesdays—he never comes. Unfolded clothes litter the floor. Chairs are piled with newspapers that date back to the Vietnam War. Pushed in a corner are boxes you meant to unpack when you moved into the house seven years ago. Stale pretzels and smelly tennis shoes are scattered under the bed.

One wife said, "I have nine books stacked on the floor by my side of the bed—they've been there for at least six months. I vacuum around them as if they're not there."

The master bedroom is often the last place to be cleaned—and decorated. A creative touch is given to the living areas, the kitchen, the children's rooms—but who will see the master bedroom? Just the two lovers.

Walk into your bedroom and take a long look. Is it a place set for passionate love? If not set the stage.

In the Song of Solomon, the king exerted great effort to prepare a luxurious bridal suite for his beloved. He even ordered cedar beams from her home country to be installed in their bedroom ceiling so his bride would feel at home (1:17). Their bed was luxuriant (1:16), probably adorned with satin and silk. A king can pay to have timber transported hundreds of miles, and creating a romantic environment is easy if servants are available to attend to your every wish. The point is, Solomon cared enough to create a place of beauty, an atmosphere conducive to passion.

We may not have servants waiting to create romantic bedrooms, but even on a limited budget we can create a haven that beckons our lover to come and revel in passionate love. Survey the scene in your bedroom and ask God (and a creative friend) where to begin the transformation. If you have the money to splurge on bedroom atmosphere, do it. If not, don't let a tight budget stop you from creating a lover's hideaway.

I (Lorraine) turned our master bedroom and bath into an English garden. A bit of floral wallpaper, a sheet made into a dust ruffle and matching curtains, and white lattice nailed to several walls began the new look. Then I wove silk ivy and roses through the lattice, added a white garden bench and an English bird cage I'd purchased at a garage sale. Finally, one coat from a ninety-nine cent can of green spray paint applied to picture frames, lamp shades, and a table completed the transformation. Total cost: $300.

Next walk into your bathroom and take a long look. According to the Unofficial U.S. Census, "The most popular sexual activity outside of actually having sex is taking showers or baths together."[3] Is your bathroom a place set for passionate love? If not, set the stage.

Today I (Linda) have a bathroom to die for. A Jacuzzi tub for two with windows overlooking the mountains. Romance is written on its walls. But our last bathroom was the ugliest thing I had ever seen. It was small beyond description. The floor had tiny tiles of pink, black, yellow, and powder blue. The tub was not only small but had dark maroon and black tile. The walls above the maroon tile were hot pink. Even the ceiling was hot pink! To top it all off, decals in pink, yellow, and powder blue adorned the cabinet. The only passion I felt in this room was for an immediate makeover.

I began a "cover-up." I covered the floor with a rug, the decals with paint, and the hot pink walls with wallpaper. Next, I traded skills with a friend, and while she made a gorgeous shower curtain and window valance to match the wallpaper, I baby-sat her children and made her dinner. A great trade. I could do nothing about the tiny tub, but many BIG memories were created in it.

Bedrooms and bathrooms can set a mood for passion. But fireplaces are a mood in themselves. If your home is blessed with a fireplace, take full advantage of it. Melinda did:

> Since we had no money for an exotic weekend away, I created a passionate hideaway at home. A friend took the children for the weekend. My only expense was the purchase of a blow-up double mattress, which I put in front of the fireplace. This became our "home away from home." My husband and I picnicked before the blazing fire, made love, shared dreams, and fell asleep in each other's arms. I hadn't realized how romantic making love and falling asleep before the glowing embers of a fire could be.

Setting the atmosphere for passion is important. And so is preparing yourself for passion.

PASSION PREPARATION

Your sense of sensuousness begins in your mind before your husband enters the room. Thinking sexually is a frame of mind, a focus. Do you allow yourself time to get into passionate focus? Remember, your mind is your most important sexual organ—so use it.

Rachel, a graphic artist who works out of her home, discovered this the hard way. "I had prepared the stage for lovemaking, told my husband to anticipate a night of passion, made his favorite dinner—all was ready except me. I worked on my project until the moment my husband walked in the door. Although the outward preparations were in place, my heart and body were set in 'project gear,' and they never really slipped into 'passionate gear.' I learned a lesson. I must prepare me, and that involves giving myself time to adopt a mind-set for passion."

"This may sound silly," JoAnne said. "What helps me to prepare is to take a bath, put on soft music and an old pair of my husband's boxer shorts.

He loves to see me in them—somehow this gets me relaxed and in the mood. I know most women feel sexy in a negligee, but for me it's boxers."

What helps you prepare your mind and body for passion? Try putting these four things in your lovemaking repertoire: fun and playfulness, tender touch, a passion exercise, and a vacation mentality.

HEY! TIME TO PLAY

In the Eskimo language, the word for sex is "laughing time." Now that's a mind-boggling thought. Would you define your lovemaking as full of fun, playfulness, and laughter? As one woman said, "We need to take the 'fore' out of foreplay and just play." Consider the playfulness of love messages.

When Lorna is in the mood for passion, she signals her husband by setting a bowl of peppermints on the nightstand by their bed. Merrilee signals she is in the mood by giving her husband not one, but three kisses in a row. Courtney lights a bedside candle when passion is on the menu. Debbie says, "Let's play a board game. I'll be the board and you play the game."

Try some of these ideas. They may seem silly, but maybe a little silliness is what's needed. Make love with your eyes closed. Make love without saying a word. Make love, whispering constantly. Make love fully clothed (don't ask "how" just try it and laugh). Go skinny dipping in a private place. Make love in a hammock. Play strip scrabble. Try different ways of kissing. It's been said that a kiss can be a comma, a question mark, or an exclamation point! Create fun trying them all.

You get the idea. Too often sex and "serious" go together. Look for ways to lighten up in the bedroom and bring back laughter, joy, and playfulness.

TENDER TOUCH IS THE TICKET

God created our bodies with a fabric of skin that responds to sensuous touch. After a few years of marriage, the way we touch each other is often reduced to one of two ways: a completely sexless, perfunctory touch (a peck on the cheek or a pat on the back), or a totally sexual touch usually limited to a few square inches of skin the dimensions of an airmail envelope. Whole kingdoms of the body and passion possibilities go unnoticed.[4]

A study at UCLA found that in order to maintain emotional and physical health, men and women needed eight to ten meaningful touches each day.[5] Touch is important not only for health but for passion. How can the passion in your heart be transmitted to your hands? Consider becoming your husband's personal masseuse. We both took a massage class so we would qualify for this activity. With a few simple lessons or a book on massage, you, too, can qualify. The nice thing is you can then encourage your husband to become your personal masseur.

One way to practice massage is to turn hair washing into a sensuous art. There is something erotic about massaging your lover's head and running your fingers through his hair. Try turning up the thermostat and leaving your nightgown and pajamas in the drawers. Fall asleep with your nude bodies touching. Sleeping nude and washing his hair are such simple pleasures. Yet these simple pleasures of touch will add a spark of passion to your love.

PRACTICE THOSE PCS

We have mentioned before your important "passion muscle": the pubococcygeal (PC) muscle. To learn where this muscle is located and how to exercise it, refer to the section in chapter 16, "Exercise Your Love Muscle."

Strengthening this muscle

- increases sensation in the pubic area and the vagina, which can increase your pleasure,
- tunes you in to your sexual desire,
- increases the intensity of orgasm,
- increases your husband's enjoyment as he can actually feel you grab his penis.[6]

VACATION VARIATIONS

Think for a moment about your most wonderful times of lovemaking. Where were you? Chances are, you were in a chalet in the mountains or a cottage at the beach. Sun, sand, sex, and no responsibilities. You were out of your ordinary routine, relaxed, and ready for spontaneity and pleasure.

How can we bottle a vacation mentality and bring it into everyday living? First, set aside time (at least three or four hours) for just the two of you to concentrate only on each other. Second, set the rules: You can talk about anything except the kids, problems at work (you get the picture). Alternate planning the time with your husband.

Possible plans to make:

A massage date. Buy a giant towel and scented massage lotion and put your expertise as a "personal masseuse" into practice.

Picnic between the sheets. Take each other and a sandwich to bed. Turn the TV off. Turn him on. Dim the lights and bring out the candles. Share something with your husband about your life that you have never told him before. Then it's his turn to share.

A motel date. This idea adds spice to your love life even if you're empty-nesters and have your house to yourselves. It's a pretend "minivacation."

If necessary, get a baby-sitter from five o'clock until midnight. Then pack a special picnic dinner and bath gift basket for your lover and spend seven whole hours alone with no phone, kids, responsibilities, or interruptions. Take something for each of the five senses (see pages 229-30) and revel in your love. It is worth the money and not much more costly than dinner and a movie. (Believe us, your husband will like it better than any movie.) One wife who took her husband on a motel minivacation said it had a trickle-down effect. Some of the sexual freedom and fun returned home with them.

A LIFELONG PASSION

You can know all the creative tips in the world but the question is, "Do you apply them? It just requires a willingness to make passion a priority. Here's a story that appeared in Ann Landers of a couple who did just that.

> Last weekend, we celebrated my parents' fiftieth wedding anniversary. This morning they left on a long awaited trip to Hawaii. They were as excited as if it were their honeymoon. When my parents married, they had only enough money for a three-day trip fifty miles from home. They made a pact that each time they made love, they would put a dollar in a special metal box and save it for a honeymoon in Hawaii for their fiftieth anniversary. Dad was a policeman, and Mom was a schoolteacher. They lived in a modest house and did all their own

repairs. Raising five children was a challenge, and sometimes, money was short. But no matter what emergency came up, Dad would not let Mom take any money out of the "Hawaii account." As the account grew, they put it in a savings account and then bought CDs.

My parents were always very much in love. I can remember Dad's coming home and telling Mom, "I have a dollar in my pocket," and she would smile at him and reply, "I know how to spend it." When each of us children married, Mom and Dad gave us a small metal box and told us their secret, which we found enchanting. All five of us are now saving for our dream honeymoons. Mom and Dad never told us how much money they had managed to save, but it must have been considerable because when they cashed in those CDs, they had enough for airfare to Hawaii plus hotel accommodations for ten days and plenty of spending money. As they told us good-bye before leaving, Dad winked and said, "Tonight, we are starting an account for Cancun. That should only take twenty-five years!"

Loving daughter in Abilene, Texas[7]

A blazing fire is not started by piling huge logs on top of one another and striking a match. The way to build a lasting fire is to start small; dry paper, bits of kindling, then small branches, and finally logs. The fire must be constantly tended to give warmth and remain bright. In the same way, the fire of your passion is built of small pieces of "kindling." Boughs of love piled on top of one another, thought upon thought, action upon action until the flame of passion blazes bright. Dear friend, it is worth the effort!

CHANGE MY HEART, O GOD

1. Check out your bedroom and bathroom atmosphere. What steps can you take to create an atmosphere more conducive to passion?

2. Pick one of the four passion possibilities listed on pages 225-7 and put it in your lovemaking repertoire this week.

LOVERS' QUARTERS INVENTORY

God built the five senses into each of us. Set the passion ablaze by becoming more aware of them and be willing to part with a few dollars to incorporate all the senses into your lovemaking.

Smell

The quickest way to induce a change in emotions or mood is through smell because the sense of smell acts more quickly on the brain than other senses.

> For you—perfume, powder, lotion (from $2 to megabucks)
>
> For the room—potpourri, scented candles (under $10); if your budget is really tight, drop a dab of cologne on your light bulbs. Then just before your lover arrives, turn on the lights and allow the scent to waft through the room, creating a pleasing aroma (free).

Sight

According to a survey conducted by the National Opinion Research Center at the University of Chicago, the second most appealing sexual act for men and women (preceded only by intercourse) was watching a partner undress.[8]

> Add to your "sight inventory" a slow, sensuous undressing (no cost—but priceless).
>
> Flickering candlelight makes everybody look better (under $10).
>
> Dimmer switch for bedroom light ($10)

Sound

Set the mood with sound sensations.

> Tabletop fountains that mimic a bubbling brook ($35 and up; available at home-improvement centers)
>
> Tapes or CDs of gentle rains, ocean waves, etc. (under $15)
>
> Tranquil Moments Plus—A small system, perfect for the bedroom that offers five built-in, digitally recorded nature sounds: waterfall, rain, ocean waves, stream, and summer night. A sixth sound soothes babies so this can be a "shared" sensory enhancer (available from Brookstone for $80).

Touch

Touch is the most effective body language. Build a repertoire that signals "Passion ahead!"

Silk or satin sheets ($50 and up)

Long slow massage (free)

A five-minute snuggle at least once a day (free)

Taste

Incorporate tingling tastes for tantalizing love.

Mint mouthwash invites lingering kisses ($2).

Your favorite drink on ice ($.50 and up)

A Hershey's Kiss on his pillow or hidden in a sweet place on your body (pennies)

How Long Does It Take to Become a Godly, Sensuous Woman?

*W*ithout exception, every one of us has the potential to become the godly, sensuous woman portrayed in Scripture, but we must realize that such a transformation takes time. Transformation means to change from the inside out and is similar to metamorphosis, the word used to picture a caterpillar as it changes into a butterfly.

We love the image of a drab, gray worm turning into a multicolored winged creature of grace and beauty, but we rarely consider the effort the worm must put forth in the process. Imagine the caterpillar reaching from within and extracting thin threads. Strand by strand, the worm weaves a cocoon around itself. Weeks pass. Externally, nothing changes, but inside the sac, the caterpillar is changing.

Like the caterpillar we, too, are transformed when we weave a cocoon of God's Word around us. We will not change overnight, but if we stay in the cocoon, we will one day emerge a glorious, free creature lifted by the wings of God to enjoy His gift of abandoned pleasure with our husbands. That's what happened for Valerie.

Valerie desired a metamorphosis in her sexual relationship with her husband. She and Bruce had been married twenty years, and while they had a good marriage, both readily described their sex life as "blah." Valerie felt she was at fault because her mind-set toward sex was so negative. Before she'd married Bruce, she'd had several unhappy sexual experiences. At seven, she'd been molested by an uncle. At twenty-one, she'd gotten pregnant by her boyfriend, Calvin. Even before she miscarried, Calvin left her. Afterward, she shut down all sexual feelings and focused her energies on growing spiritually.

Valerie attended a Bible study we offered on the sexual relationship in marriage. "I've put off growing in this area of my life for too long," she said. "Show me what to do." I (Linda) asked Valerie if she would be willing to meet with me weekly and accept "assignments" that would include reading chapters from this book, memorizing Scripture, and writing a journal. She agreed. The journal that follows is hers. She gave us permission to share it in hopes that what she is learning might encourage you.

VALERIE'S JOURNAL

July 25
I met with Linda this afternoon. God, You were so present in our conversation, so near as we prayed. We both sensed we were on holy ground, that You were giving us glimpses of Your mind and heart as it relates to sex. Lord, You know that sex is a burden for me, but I want to grow in my thinking because I want to honor You and honor my husband.

August 3
I just read the chapter called "How Can I Be Godly *and* Sensuous," and I realized the reason I don't enjoy sex much is because I don't give myself permission to receive sensuous love. I dated many men in the ten years before I met Bruce, and it seems most of that time was spent fighting guys off (You warned me, Lord, about dating guys who weren't Christians, but I didn't listen). No. No. No. I must have said the word a thousand times. When I met Calvin, I said yes. I knew what I was doing was wrong. I paid a hefty price too. After we broke up, I stayed away from sex. Then Bruce and I married, and suddenly I was supposed to always say yes and change my thinking to *This is right*. I tried, but something in me said that enjoying sex *too much* was still wrong.

August 10
My sensuous side feels like a prisoner, locked up and confined. Poor Bruce. He's been so patient with me. It's as if he has this wonderful room in his

life labeled "intimate pleasures with my wife" that he's never been able to go into because I've locked the door and misplaced the key. As a result, his sexual growth has been stunted along with mine.

I want to say, "I'm ready, honey. God has given us the key. Let's unlock the door together." But I'm afraid. It's so foreign to me. I don't feel like anything behind that door belongs to me, or that it will fit. But God, what's in that room are things you want me to put on, things You designed just for me. It will fit. I will look beautiful in it. My husband will be so thrilled with what I put on. But I have to believe these things by faith because everything inside insists what is behind that door is for someone else, not me.

August 12
This week I read chapter 3 about my mind. I'd never realized how important my mind was in sex. I definitely need a mind transplant. I'm going to memorize two verses from the Song of Solomon. I hope it will help.

August 17
Linda challenged me to pick one thing to do this week to enhance my lovemaking with Bruce. After reading the chapter "How Can Sex Go from Boring to Sizzling?" I decided I would try to be more verbal in our lovemaking since right now, I say nothing. This may seem like a stroll in the park to someone else. But to me it's scary. What if I sound stupid? Can I say things I don't really feel? Can I behave in a way that, for me, feels unnatural?

God, the truth is, I don't see myself as a sensuous woman, but You do. My husband does. I'm going to trust, God, that as I act upon what I have purposed to do You will help me see myself through Your eyes. I love You, Father, and I love my husband. I place myself in Your hands, claiming Your promise in Philippians 1:6: You who have begun a good work in me *will* be faithful to complete it.

August 19
Yesterday was one of the most beautiful times of making love we've ever had. I spent two hours preparing myself and the bathroom. Candles and perfume to delight the nose, a bubbling fountain and piano music for the ears, cheese sticks and egg rolls for the mouth, flowers and bubbles for the

eyes (not to mention a see-through teddy). My husband was *very* happy. He contributed sparkling cider and fresh flowers. We spent two hours enjoying it all and each other. I'd heard before about couples spending hours making love and wondered what in the world they did. I'm beginning to see.

I read the first part of my journal to Bruce as we soaked in the bathtub. I needed to express my doubts and feelings of failure to him. He was so tender with me. I know he appreciates the effort I'm putting forth even though he doesn't say so. I was more verbally expressive to him. I felt a bit silly, but he loved it.

August 21

I find myself thinking at the oddest times about the verses I'm memorizing—while pushing the cart in the grocery store and singing in church. God, please use your Word to change my view of sex.

August 22

Thank You, Father, for changing me as only Your Spirit can. Please continue Your work in me. I still have far to go. I praise You for a patient husband like Bruce and a faithful, inspiring friend like Linda. They, too, will be Your instruments for my growth.

August 28

I hate hormones. I hate PMS. And I really hate sex. What is all the fuss about anyway? It seems to me a pretty weird way for two people to be united. Why, God, did you make us so different? I've had enough of sex, and Bruce can't get enough of it. I have NO desire. Zero. I pigged out at the barbecue, and I feel so fat I am repulsed at the thought of his touching me. Why, oh why, did I commit to grow in this area of my life?

September 1

The kids are back in school, so it's time for me to get back in the groove of life. In addition to the sixty regular items on my to-do list, I added "diet," "clean the garage," and "sex." I had to put sex on my to-do list, otherwise I'd never consider it at all. God, will sex always be work for me? Will it always be something I have to force myself to think about and force myself to do? I'm committed to grow in this area, and I will . . . I will! But can't You give me some desire? Please?

September 2

I forced myself to initiate sex because I knew Bruce was about ready to explode. He needs the sexual release because he is under so much tension at work. It was fine. I think I've been making myself too performance-oriented and I need to relax a bit and know that a splash of perfume, some nice music, and a quickie are fine now and then.

September 16

God, there is hope! Last night was quite possibly the best sex we've ever had in twenty years of marriage. I pulled out all the stops: new nightgown, candles, soft music, our favorite beverage. I spent an hour in the shower, splashing on fragrant jells, washing my hair, and shaving my legs. Afterward I painted my fingernails and toenails, then rubbed every part of my body with lotion. I looked good, smelled good, felt good—and IT was good.

My husband smirked over coffee, "Sure was fun last night." He called me from work and said, "Sure enjoyed last night." What made last night so special? I was different. I didn't feel so "bound up." I relaxed and moved with him. I talked more, objected less. I let him do things I usually feel squeamish about. I'm growing. Reading again the chapter on "How Can I Be Godly *and* Sensuous?" really helped. I've been acutely aware in the last few months that I have definitely put sensuous feelings in one box and God in another, never allowing the two to mingle. Because I allowed myself to have sex before marriage, and because I knew God disapproved of that, the only way I could keep having sex with my boyfriend AND keep growing in my relationship with God was to separate the two.

Reading the part in the Bible about God standing over Shulamith and Solomon and blessing their sexual union helped me integrate the spiritual and the sensuous. I think that's what happened last night: the beginnings of these two passions coming together. I still have a long way to go, but there is growth! Thank you, God.

October 12

Ten days ago I was in a car accident. My body feels like it's been run over by a semi instead of being sideswiped by a Toyota. I've got a broken toe, a bruised left hip, and whiplash. Last night for the first time since the accident we made love. The only way I could get comfortable was to lie flat on my back, shove a pillow under my left hip, and dangle my right leg halfway off the side of the bed. We didn't do much kissing since I can't move my neck. Bruce held back for fear he would hurt me, even though I told him I was okay. It did hurt, but it wasn't unbearable.

I told Linda about it, and she suggested I try some alternate things, like just bringing pleasure to him while we are standing up in the shower. The warm water pounding on my neck would feel good, and Bruce wouldn't complain. I was embarrassed to tell her I'd never done anything like that before. Instead of making me feel prudish, she affirmed me for being willing to try something new.

October 27

Bruce made partner at his law firm today! This is something he's been working toward for years. There were lots of things we could do to celebrate: go out to eat, call friends, go to a movie. But I knew what would mean more to him than anything: an afternoon alone with me in a sexy bodysuit. If I were the one celebrating a big achievement, I'd want a big party with food and friends. But Bruce just wanted me—all of me—and my focus on him and his body. So that's what I did. It felt good to set my selfishness aside and think of him and his needs. As we lay on the bed afterward, enjoying the warmth of each other's bodies, he said, "I wish all couples could know the happiness we enjoy together."

Whenever he thinks of making partner, he'll remember me, his *true* partner.

November 3

It's been awful. Bruce's brother was killed yesterday. A drunk driver. Bruce was distraught. At 2 A.M., sleep eluded us as we both anguished over the turn of events. I wished I could take away some of his pain. Then I remembered that I had read one of the reasons God gave the gift of sex was for comfort. Even though my neck and shoulders were aching (the whiplash hangs on), I comforted my husband with my body. I rubbed the tension from his shoulders, then gave myself to him. His release was so intense he cried. At last, he could sleep. I have not always rightly viewed sex as God's gift, but at that moment, I realized no other gift I could have given could have meant more.

November 15

I decided to take another step forward in being more verbal during our lovemaking. Last night I actually "made sounds" when I came. I told Bruce how good he'd made me feel. You'd have thought I gave him a million dollars. I feel so humbled, God, that such a little thing makes him so happy. Why has it taken me twenty years to realize this?

November 26

Linda asked me if I would be willing to try an idea in which Bruce and I would spend several hours making love. (See the sealed envelope at the back of the book.) I couldn't imagine what we would do that would take so long, but I told her I'd give it a try. Linda was so encouraging. She said, "Valerie, three months ago you would never have tried this. You are growing."

December 2

I pinned an invitation to an evening of "Gourmet Delight" on a sexy teddy and put it in Bruce's car. He called me the moment he got to work and said, "I don't know what you're up to, but it sure sounds fun." He seemed so pleased that I would go to so much trouble for him.

December 4

I got the kids to the baby-sitter and soaked in the tub for an hour and read Song of Solomon in order to prepare my body and my mind for our special night. When Bruce walked in the door, he heard Kenny G. playing the saxophone and smelled inviting aromas coming from the kitchen.

I took him by the hand and led him to the den, where I handed him a virgin strawberry margarita and a note that said, "Anything above the neck is permissible." I was surprised at how long we lingered over our drinks!

Then I led him from room to room where we enjoyed tasty delights and lots of touching. By the time we got to the last course, I was the one urging him to hurry up and eat so we could get to dessert—which was me!

What a riot! In twenty years of marriage we've never had so much fun during lovemaking. Bruce says Gourmet Delight is now his favorite dish, and he wants to have it at least once a week. Thank you, God, for showing me how much fun making love can be.

December 31

It is New Year's Eve—time to set goals for the coming year. I've set three for myself in growing to become a sensuous wife to Bruce. I'm going to

- make our sexual relationship and my sexual growth a matter of daily prayer,
- memorize one scripture about sex each month,
- try one of the creative lovemaking suggestions found in Linda and Lorraine's book once a month.

It feels good to set goals. I'm growing. I pray You are pleased, God. I know my husband is!

START TODAY

God is weaving the strands of His Word around Valerie's heart. She is beginning to emerge as a sexual butterfly—free, lifted by the wings of God to enjoy His gift of abandoned pleasure with her husband.

Where you are today? Are you going forward in the goal of becoming a godly and sensuous wife or still thinking about it? Dear Friend, don't wait. Perhaps it would be helpful for you to keep a journal to record your steps forward (and backward) as Valerie did. God is faithful. He loves you with an everlasting love. His mercies are new every morning. Write them down. In light of eternity, becoming a godly and sensuous wife will take no time at all.

CHANGE MY HEART, O GOD

1. Keep your own journal. (Make sure it has a lock on it or it is hidden is a safe place.)

2. Determine one new thing you'd like to try this week in your lovemaking.

3. Find a trustworthy friend who will pray for you and encourage you to grow to become the godly and sensuous wife of Scripture.

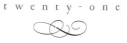

twenty-one

The Granddaddy of All Questions:
(hint: look in the mirror)

What is it like to make love to me?

What words characterize you as a lover? Warm? Joyful? Sensuous? Creative? Aggressive? Fun? Or words like boring, unimaginative, and inhibited? Ask God to help you see the truth. Get behind your husband's eyes and see yourself as he sees you. Take paper and pen and write a description of yourself as a lover.

Next, consider being brave and asking your husband the following question: What can I do to become your dream lover?

When you ask your husband this question, you are saying, "Honey, I long to grow as a sensuous woman. I long to become all you've ever dreamed of in a lover." Can you think of any gift he would rather receive? And once you've been brave enough to ask this question, you are committed to moving forward as a godly and sensuous wife. That is exciting!

To help you move ahead, we have included one practical suggestion in the sealed envelope at the end of the book. So . . . open the "Intimate Secret," and continue on the journey to becoming a godly and sensuous wife.

Twelve Weeks to Becoming a Godly and Sensuous Wife

*D*ear Friend,

Many women read a book such as this one and excitedly think, "Yes! I want to apply these truths in my marriage." But as the days pass, their enthusiasm and commitment wane because they fail to search the Scriptures and allow God's Spirit to work lasting change in their lives. We applaud you for taking that extra step—for being willing to immerse yourself in God's Word so that the new thoughts in your mind will become reality in your actions. We pray that in the weeks to come you will look back and say, "I'm so glad I did this study." We know your husband will be thankful!

PURPOSE

The purpose of this twelve-week study is to saturate your heart and mind with God's Word so that your sexual attitudes may be conformed to God's attitude about sex. You will need a copy of this book, a Bible, and a notebook in which to record your answers. You can do the study on your own, but we think you will find it encouraging to discuss what you are learning with other women.

Because of the highly sensitive subject matter in this book, we have selected for the Bible study only those topics that lend themselves to group discussion. If subjects like sexual abuse, abortion, or pornography affect you, please don't overlook them just because they are not part of the group study. Instead, reread the chapters and do the "Change My Heart, O God" section at the end. Unless God leads you otherwise, we would encourage you not to share these details with your group but instead to talk with a

Christian counselor or a mature, godly friend who has knowledge about the issues that impact you.

GUIDELINES

If you are joining with other women for this study, we encourage you to ask each woman to commit to the following guidelines during your initial meeting.

1. Keep the focus of the study centered on God. Share what you are learning about God and His perspective on the sexual relationship or what God is personally teaching you.

2. Under no circumstances should you share with others intimate details about your sexual relationship with your husband. No one should ever be able to visualize you and your husband in bed. It would be wise to reassure your husband of your commitment to keep your sexual relationship private.

3. Start and end your time in prayer. You'll find that your time together is much more effective when you invite the Holy Spirit to work in your hearts.

When we offered a similar study at our church, we repeatedly heard comments like:

> "Thanks to this study, my sexual relationship with my husband is better than it's ever been."

> "Because I was sexually abused, I viewed sex as dirty. Now I see it as holy."

> "I understand for the first time that God intended for the sexual and spiritual to intertwine, not to be separate."

We pray your group will enjoy similar revelations. May God richly bless your time in His Word as you seek to become your husband's "Shulamith."

Linda & Lorraine

Linda and Lorraine

lesson one

What Does God Think About Sex?

Read chapter 1: What Does God Think About Sex?

1. Write a short paragraph describing how you first learned about sex. How did this influence your thinking about the sexual relationship? What other "voices" have influenced your thinking over the years? Be prepared to talk about these in your group.

2. As Christians, we want to listen to the one true voice—God's voice. According to chapter 1, what does God say about why He gave us the gift of sex? Do any of the six reasons surprise you? If so, which ones and why?

    Comfort - it feels like betrayal of the grief to enjoy sex.

3. In Genesis 4:1 (KJV), Adam "knew" Eve. The Hebrew word for intercourse means "to know." In what way does the sexual relationship give you special knowledge about your husband? *He isn't the sure, strong minded manager - just a man needing love!*

4. In 2 Samuel 12:24 when Bathsheba was grieving the death of her son, David comforted her with sexual intercourse. In what circumstances could you give the gift of sex as a comfort to your husband? *When he feels overwhelmed w/ stuff @ factory. - When he feels betrayed by a friend or worker - he has been criticized*

5. Read Genesis 2:24 and Ephesians 5:31-32. Describe in your own words what it means to be "one flesh" with your husband.

6. Read Proverbs 5. What solution do verses 15-19 offer to the questions posed in the rest of the chapter?

7. Memorize Proverbs 5:18-19. Write the verses on paper, then rewrite them as a prayer of thanksgiving to God for the gift of pleasure.

8. This week, plan a special evening with your husband to focus on one of the six reasons God gave the gift of sex.

9. Write a paragraph you could give to your daughter or to another woman describing God's viewpoint on sex.

How Can I Be Godly *and* Sensuous?

Read chapter 2: How Can I Be Godly and Sensuous?

1. Read the Song of Solomon (also called the Song of Songs) through in one sitting. As you read, ask God to speak to you about who you are as a sensuous woman.

2. In what ways do you tend to separate your spirituality from your sensuousness? What circumstances or attitudes have contributed to this thinking?

3. In Song of Solomon 5:1, Solomon and Shulamith have just enjoyed the ecstasy of sexual intimacy. Suddenly God appears beside their bed and pronounces His blessing upon the couple. Imagine your honeymoon night and God pronouncing His blessing upon you and your husband. Rewrite Song of Solomon 5:1 in your own words, using you and your husband as the two lovers.

4. Memorize Romans 11:36 (TLB): "For everything comes from God alone. Everything lives by his power, and everything is for his glory. To him be glory evermore." As you repeat the verse, thank God that "everything" includes your sexuality.

5. Shulamith was responsive, adventurous, uninhibited, expressive, and sensuous. Find at least three verses to confirm each of these characteristics. Write out the verses under the following headings:

    a. How was Shulamith responsive?

    b. How was Shulamith adventurous?

    c. How was Shulamith uninhibited?

    d. How was Shulamith expressive?

    e. How was Shulamith sensuous?

6. Which of these five characteristics comes naturally to you? Which is most difficult? Select one area you'd like to work on this week and determine a concrete action you will take. (Example: "I need to be more expressive. This week when we make love, I will verbalize to my husband what feels good.")

7. What did you learn about God in the Song of Solomon? What did you learn about yourself?

lesson   three

How Do I Shift into Sexual Gear?

Read chapter 3: How Do I Shift into Sexual Gear?

1. Memorize the first portion of Romans 12:2: "Do not be conformed to this world, but be transformed by the renewing of your mind."

2. In this chapter, you were asked to picture your mind as a flower bed, with weeds representing wrong sexual thoughts and flowers representing God's thoughts. Using this image, write a detailed description of your flower bed.

3. Read Psalm 139:1-3, Psalm 26:1-2, Isaiah 55:8-9, and Daniel 2:22-23. According to these verses, why is inviting God to search your mind a key step in developing an accurate picture of your flower bed?

4. What warning is issued in Romans 1:28 to those who allow themselves to think wrong thoughts? According to Romans 1:24-27, what indecent sexual acts result from a depraved mind?

5. On a separate sheet of paper, make a list of the "weeds" (wrong thoughts) you want to uproot. Spend time in prayer asking God to remove these weeds. After you have given your "weeds" to God, rip up your paper and throw it in the trash or burn it.

6. Deuteronomy 11:18 tells us to fix God's words in our minds. How do we do this? What instruction is provided in Romans 8:5,11; Philippians 4:8-9; Ephesians 4:22-23,29; and Psalm 119:11?

7. List at least three "flower seeds" (scriptural thoughts about sex) you feel God wants you to plant in your mind.

8. In the Song of Solomon 5:10-16, Shulamith lingers on a mental picture of her husband's naked body. Why do you think God included this in His holy Word? In what ways does Shulamith allow her mind to drift in her daydreaming? In what ways does she restrain her thoughts?

9. First Peter 1:13 says we are to "gird up the loins of [our] minds" (KJV). Second Corinthians 10:5 tells us to take "every thought captive to the obedience of Christ." Based on these verses and the mental disciplines we've already discussed, write a step-by-step plan for managing your sexual thoughts. How do you think following this plan will change your sexual mind-set?

How Can I Relate When He's a Microwave and I'm a Crockpot?

Read chapter 4: How Can I Relate When He's a Microwave and I'm a Crockpot?

1   Read Genesis 2:4-25, and make a list of the created differences between man and woman. (You might want to refer to our list on pages 34-5.) What do you think God's purpose was in creating these differences?

2.   Read Genesis 2:18. In what ways are you physically, emotionally, spiritually, and sexually a helper for your husband? List at least six.

3.   When God brought Eve to Adam, Adam said, "This is now bone of my bones, and flesh of my flesh" (Genesis 2:23). The Living Bible translates Adam's enthusiasm for Eve as, "This is it!" Write your own translation of this verse. How does Adam's "Wow!" response reinforce the idea that God made men visually oriented and physically responsive?

4.   Read Genesis 1:26-27. Why do you think *both* male and female are required to reflect God's image? What attributes does your husband possess that you lack? What attributes do you possess that he lacks? How do your differences reveal a more complete picture of God?

5.   Read Genesis 2:24. In what ways can physical intimacy heal division?

6.   Write a prayer thanking God for the differences in your marriage and praising Him for His gift of sex in which you can experience oneness.

Couple exercise (not for group discussion):
If your husband is willing, read through this chapter together and discuss what is true for you as a couple. Then share with each other how you would fill in the blank in the following question: "My favorite part of lovemaking is _____."

lesson   five

What Do I Do When I Don't Want to Do It?

Read chapter 5: What Do I Do When I Don't Want to Do It?

1. Three women gave these descriptions of their attitudes about sex:

    a. "Sex is a thankless chore. Most of the time, I could do without it."

    b. "When my husband signals me he wants to make love and I'm not in the mood, I find some excuse so we don't have to."

    c. "When I don't want to do it, I pray and ask God to help me rise above my personal excuses and minister to my husband."

    Write a short paragraph that describes your own sexual attitude.

2. Write in your own words a paraphrase of 1 Corinthians 7:3-5.

3. How does it affect your view of sex to realize that "duty" means the payment of a debt that is owed?

4. How might your attitude change if you viewed sexual intimacy as a "gift exchange"?

5. Write a paragraph describing how you would share the principles of need, authority, and faithfulness (as detailed in this chapter) with your daughter or friend.

6. Read Philippians 2:3-5. How does this passage apply to your sexual relationship?

7. Attitude is defined as an inward feeling expressed by outward behavior. In Philippians 2:5-11, we are told to have the same attitude as Jesus Christ.

    a. What was Christ's attitude?

    b. How does this apply to the sexual relationship when the wife isn't "in the mood"?

8. What does 1 Corinthians 7:33-34 identify as one responsibility of a married woman? How does this apply to you?

9. Memorize 1 Corinthians 7:4.

Where Can I Go to Buy a New Body?

Read chapter 6: Where Can I Go to Buy a New Body?

1. Three important concepts were discussed in this chapter: (1) Accept the body God gave you. (2) Develop the beauty of a sensuous wife. (3) Be responsible with your "temple." Write three short paragraphs describing how you would teach these concepts to your daughter or to another woman.

2. List three ways a wife's feelings about her body affect her ability to be a creative lover.

3. Write Psalm 139:14 on a sheet of paper, and tape it to your mirror. Then stand in front of the bathroom mirror naked. Review your body from the top of your head to the tip of your toes, and praise God that you are "fearfully and wonderfully made."

4. Memorize Psalm 139:14.

5. Write a short description of your reaction to each of the follow statements:
    a. "It's better to be sensuous than to have a perfect '10' body."
    b. "Nothing transcends the traditional definitions of beauty like the face and body of a passionately aroused woman."
    c. "There is a natural beauty that emanates from a woman who has done the most with what she has and learned to use her body to delight and entice her husband."

6. Read about the undisciplined woman in Proverbs 6:6-11; 24:30-34; 26:13-16. Ask God if any of these descriptions apply to you. If they do, write one action you will begin this week to better care for your "temple."

7. Read Proverbs 24:30-33. What does it mean to you personally to see, reflect on, and receive instruction? How does this apply to your care of your body?

8. Reread the five suggestions listed under the heading "Learn from What You See" on pages 62-3. Pick one of these suggestions to put into practice this week. Write a paragraph detailing your plan of application.

9. What did you learn about God this week? What did you learn about yourself? Write a prayer to God expressing what you learned. If you feel comfortable, share your prayer with your group.

How Can I Get over the Guilt of Past Sexual Sin?

Read chapter 8: How Can I Get over the Guilt of Past Sexual Sin?

1. Guilt is the breaking of a law that requires a penalty. Shame is the painful emotion that accompanies guilt. Genesis 2:25 says, "The man and his wife were both naked and were not ashamed." Read Genesis 3:1-12.

    a. At what point did Adam and Eve experience guilt?

    b. When did they feel shame?

    c. What did these feelings cause them to do?

2. Hebrews 9:22 says, "Without shedding of blood there is no forgiveness [of sin]."

    a. According to Genesis 3:21, how was blood shed to cover Adam and Eve's sin?

    b. Read Hebrews 9:13, Ephesians 1:7, and Revelation 1:5. How was blood shed to cover our sin?

3. Read 1 John 1:8-10 and Psalm 32:1-5. According to these verses, what happens when we fail to acknowledge our sin? What can we expect when we confess our sin?

4. Look up the words *correct* and *condemn* in the dictionary. Read Proverbs 3:11-12, John 8:10-11, 1 Peter 5:8, and Revelation 12:10. Who corrects us and why? Who condemns us and why?

5. Read about the adulteress who was forgiven in Luke 7:36-50. What was Jesus' attitude toward this woman? Who condemned her? Who corrected her? Why is Jesus able to extend forgiveness for sins?

6. Go to Jesus now. Confess your sin and allow Him to extend forgiveness to you. According to Hebrews 10:19-22, how should you approach God now that you are forgiven?

7. Read through the "Change My Heart, O God" section on pages 89-90. Spend some time alone with God, meditating on Psalms 51 and 52 and working through the practical applications.

I'm Attracted to Another Man! Help?

Read chapter 9: I'm Attracted to Another Man! Help?

1. We stated that 90 percent of the women we surveyed in church leadership and at a women's retreat said they had faced sexual temptation. Does this statistic surprise you? Why or why not?

2. Read Genesis 3:1-8. Eve's temptation progressed through the three stages described in chapter 9: *Temptation, Contemplation,* and *Activation.* Describe her actions and choices in each stage.

3. Read Genesis 3:8-24. List the consequences that occurred because of Eve's failure to say no to temptation. How did Eve's choice affect others? If you give in to your temptations, who would be impacted by your choices and how?

4. Read Matthew 4:1-11. "Then Jesus was led up by the Spirit into the wilderness to be tempted by the devil" (verse 1). Why would the Spirit permit Jesus to be tempted? What positive benefits can temptation produce?

5. How did Jesus fight temptation in Matthew 4:1-11? Who was being tempted in Luke 22:39-46 and why? What do these passages show you about how you can fight temptation?

6. Hebrews 2:18 says, "For since He Himself was tempted in that which He has suffered, He is able to come to the aid of those who are tempted." How can Jesus help when you face temptation?

7. Read through the six "escape routes" described on pages 97-101. Write down several escape plans you will put in place today to help you resist temptation in the future.

8. Memorize 1 Corinthians 10:13: "No temptation has overtaken you but such as is common to man; and God is faithful, who will not allow you to be tempted beyond what you are able, but with the temptation will provide the way of escape also, that you may be able to endure it."

How Can I Remain Faithful in a Faithless World?

Read chapter 10: How Can I Remain Faithful in a Faithless World?

1. The word *covenant,* used approximately three hundred times in the Word of God, refers to a binding agreement in which the parties involved promise to fulfill certain vows. Write out the vows you made on your wedding day. (We strongly urge you to spend time reminiscing by reviewing your wedding photos, videos, or any other memorabilia you have of that day.)

2. In this chapter we said that faithfulness in marriage is more than the *absence* of an affair or the absence of a divorce document. Faithfulness involves the *presence* of the love, devotion, honor, loyalty, and encouragement we vowed at the altar. Write a short paragraph describing how you are—or are not—being faithful to the vows you made on your wedding day.

3. Read Numbers 30:1-2, Deuteronomy 23:21-23, Ecclesiastes 5:4-5. Write in your own words what God says in these verses about keeping your vows.

4. Read Romans 12:3, 1 Peter 3:8-9, Colossians 3:13-14, Philippians 2:1-5, and Psalm 62:8. Make a list of the attitudes found in these verses that will help you to fulfill your vows.

5. God says, "I hate divorce." What are some reasons given in Malachi 2:13-16 for this strong statement?

6. According to Matthew 19:8, what is one of the main causes of divorce? List at least three ways a vital sexual relationship with your husband can help to keep your hearts tender toward each other.

7. What encouragement is offered in Proverbs 5:15-19? Determine one thing you will do this week to help your husband be exhilarated with your love.

8. Talk with a couple who has been married twenty years or more and whose relationship you respect. Ask how they got through difficult times in their marriage, and encourage them to share any advice or marriage tips that have helped them. (Consider inviting them for dinner so your husband can benefit from the interview too.) Write a summary of what you learned, and share it with your study group.

9. Bring one of your wedding pictures to share with the group, then spend time praying for each of the marriages represented.

How Can Sex Go from Boring to Sizzling?

Read chapter 15: How Can Sex Go from Boring to Sizzling?

1. Using a dictionary, write out the definitions of *boring* and *creative*.

2. In what areas are you praised for your creativity?

3. Shulamith used fragrance and words creatively in her love relationship with Solomon. She also used her body in provocative ways. Another woman in Scripture used these creative means for evil. Read about the adulterous woman in Proverbs 5–7, and record how she used creativity:

    a. with her words
    b. with her body

4. Give at least three reasons you think the man followed after the woman described in Proverbs 5–7.

5. What is the answer to the creative snares of the adulteress in Proverbs 5:15-19?

6. Write a modern paraphrase of Proverbs 5:15-19.

7. Personalize Proverbs 5:19 by writing it as a prayer to God.

8. In this chapter we quote Stephen Covey's philosophy: "The key to creativity is to begin with the end in view." Write a paragraph describing who you want to be as a lover five years from now. Then list at least three things you will do in the next month to help you grow as a godly, sensuous wife.

l e s s o n   e l e v e n
How Can I Recapture the Passion?

Read chapter 19: How Can I Recapture the Passion?

1. One source defines passion as "a compelling, intense feeling or emotion; love, ardent affection, amorous desire." The Hebrew word translated as *passion* in Today's English Version or the New Revised Standard Version of Song of Solomon 8:6-7 is often used in the Old Testament to describe the passion of God. Other Bible versions translate this word as *jealousy* or *zeal.* Read 2 Kings 19:31, Isaiah 9:7, Isaiah 37:32, and Jeremiah 31:3. From these verses, write a definition of the passion of God.

2. Read Song of Solomon 8:6-7.
    a. What do you learn about God in these verses?
    b. What do you learn about the passionate love between a husband and wife?

3. The German philosopher Goethe said, "Things which matter most must never be at the mercy of things which matter least." Your love relationship with your husband is important to God and to you. List five ways you can make passion a priority in your marriage.

4. Your sensuousness begins in your mind before your husband enters the room. Thinking sexually is a frame of mind, a focus. List three things you can do that will help you prepare your mind and heart for passion.

5. Reread the section "Set an Atmosphere for Passion" on pages 222-4. Check out the atmosphere in your bedroom and bathroom. List several steps you can take to create an atmosphere more conducive to passion.

6. Reread "A Lifelong Passion" on pages 227-8. How does this story make you feel? What practical actions can you take to ignite and sustain a lifelong passion with your husband?

7. Pick one of the four passion possibilities listed on page 225, and add it to your lovemaking repertoire this week.

8. Write a prayer thanking God for His passionate love for you and the passionate love He desires for you to have with your husband.

lesson   twelve

A Time of Praise

For eleven weeks you have studied God's perspective on the sexual relationship. Week twelve is a time to offer thanksgiving and to celebrate what God has revealed to you.

Thanksgiving (on your own, prior to meeting)
Start each day by thanking God for something He has taught you. In addition, complete the following assignments:

1. Review material from the last eleven weeks. Write several paragraphs expressing what you have learned *about God*. Praise God for how clearly He has expressed His views on the sexual relationship in Scripture.

2. Write several paragraphs expressing what you have learned *about yourself* or *your sexual relationship*. Thank God for what He has revealed about your attitudes and actions.

3. Prepare something to share with your group during your celebration time. (See suggestions under *Celebration*.)

Celebration (group time)
Your time of celebration will be during your final group time. Decide in advance how this time will look (consider a potluck at someone's home). Allow time for each woman to share how this study has impacted her view of the sexual relationship. Here are six suggestions:

1. Read something you wrote for an assignment.

2. Write a song or poem thanking God for what He has shown you.

3. Write a letter to your daughter (daughter-in-law, granddaughter) expressing what you have learned.

4. Make an acrostic using a word like *intimacy*, or cite from memory a passage of Scripture that has been meaningful to you.

5. Draw a graph that shows how you have grown.

6. Paint a picture of the new flower bed in your mind.

End with a time of worship and prayer, celebrating what God has done.

ADDITIONAL RESOURCES

WHERE CAN YOU GET MORE HELP FOR POST-ABORTION
SYNDROME?

Organizations

Care Net

109 Carpenter Drive, Suite 100, Sterling, VA 20164

(703) 478-5661

E-mail: Carenet@erols.com

The organization will help you find the crisis-pregnancy center nearest you.
These centers offer courses or material in post-abortion healing.

Women Exploited by Abortion (WEBA)

P.O. Box 278, Dawson, TX 76639

They have chapters in fifty states designed to help women who suffer the lingering effects of abortion.

National Memorial for the Unborn

6230 Vance Road, Chattanooga, TN 37421

(423) 954-9552

Contact them to purchase a plaque in memory of your child, which is placed
on a memorial wall.

Bible Studies

Women in Ramah: A Post Abortion Bible Study, a women's study
Call Care Net, (703) 478-5661

In His Image, a study for men and women
Call Open Arms, (719) 573-5790

Video

> *After the Choice,* a video of thirteen women who have had abortions. Call Concerned Women for America, 800-527-9600.

Fiction

> Francine Rivers, *Atonement Child* (Wheaton, Ill.: Tyndale, 1997).

WHERE CAN YOU GET MORE HELP BATTLING PORNOGRAPHY?

Organizations

> **National Coalition Against Pornography**
> 800 Compton Road, Suite 9224; Cincinnati, Ohio 45231
> (513) 521-6227
>
> Provides training resources, videos, audio cassettes, and research material on pornography

> **Pure Life Ministries**
> P. O. Box 410, Dry Ridge, KY 41035
> (606) 824-4444
> Offers intensive counseling and Bible study

Books

> Laurie Hall, *An Affair of the Mind,* (Colorado Springs: Focus on the Family Publishing, 1996). One woman's story of her courageous fight against pornography in her home.

> Tom Minnery, *Pornography: A Human Tragedy* (Wheaton, Ill.: Tyndale, 1987). Provides a thoughtful social commentary of the effect of pornography on our nation.

> Dr. Harry Schaumburg, *False Intimacy: Understanding the Struggle of Sexual Addictions* (Colorado Springs: NavPress, 1992). Offers excellent insight into sexual addictions.

WHERE CAN YOU GET MORE HELP FOR OVERCOMING THE PAIN OF SEXUAL ABUSE?

Following are additional resources you may find helpful:

Tapes

"Healing Childhood Traumas," the story of Stephanie Fast. Contact Focus on the Family at (719) 531-3400 and ask for two tapes, CS298.

Books

Dr. Dan Allender, *The Wounded Heart* (Colorado Springs: NavPress, 1990*)*.

Dr. Harry Schaumburg, *False Intimacy: Understanding the Struggle of Sexual Addictions* (Colorado Springs: NavPress, 1992).

Organizations

Wounded Heart Ministries, Dr. Dan Allender. Offers workshops around the country as well as a newsletter. Call Western Seminary at (888) 977-2002 and ask for information.

Freedom in Christ Ministries, Dr. Neil Anderson, 10 West Dry Creek Circle, Littleton, CO, 80120; (303) 730-4211. Offers seminars around the country on how to be free from the chains of the past and to live free in Christ.

Counseling

Call the Rape Abuse Incest National Network Hot Line at 1-800-656-HOPE. You can speak to an advocate who will help you find resources in your area.

Call (719) 531-3400, or write Focus on the Family, Colorado Springs, CO, 80995-7451. Limited telephone counseling available. Also, the correspondence department can suggest helpful resources.

New Life Clinics offer counseling and group therapy. Call (800) NEW-LIFE, and ask for the clinic nearest you.

Contact a local pastor and ask for therapists trained in biblical counseling for sexual-abuse victims.

Notes

Dear Reader . . .

1. Ann Landers, *Colorado Springs Gazette*, 23 November 1997, Lifestyle sec., 4.

2. Steve Marshall, "Harassment Makes Skies Not So Friendly," *USA Today*, 12 June 1998, sec. A, 4.

Chapter 1: What Does God Think About Sex?

1. Eric Fuchs, *Sexual Desire and Love* (New York: Seabury Press, 1983), 108.

2. Mary Ann Mayo, *A Christian Guide to Sexual Counseling* (Grand Rapids, Mich.: Zondervan, 1987), 28.

3. Tim Stafford, *Sexual Chaos* (Downers Grove, Ill.: InterVarsity, 1993), 37.

4. Mike Mason, *The Mystery of Marriage* (Portland, Ore.: Multnomah, 1985), 124.

5. Linda Dillow, *Creative Counterpart* (Nashville: Nelson, 1977), 169.

Chapter 2: How Can I Be Godly and Sensuous?

1. Dan B. Allender and Tremper Longman III, *Intimate Allies* (Wheaton, Ill.: Tyndale, 1995), 233-4.

2. Allender and Longman, *Intimate Allies*, 215.

3. William R. Newell, *Romans: Verse by Verse* (Chicago: Moody, 1938), 444.

4. Conversation with Vonette Bright, 19 September 1998. Used by permission.

5. Hebrew scholars commonly give the name "Shulamith" to Solomon's bride. The name means "a female resident of the town of Shunem." G. W. Bromley, ed., *The International Standard Encyclopedia*, vol. 4 (Grand Rapids, Mich.: Eerdmans, 1988), 497.

6. Richard G. Moulton, "Lyric Idyll: Solomon's Song," *The Literary Study of the Bible* (London: Isbiter & Co., Limited, 1903), 207-24.

7. Allender and Longman, *Intimate Allies*, 252.

8. Allender and Longman, *Intimate Allies*, 252.

Chapter 3: How Do I Shift into Sexual Gear?

1. Douglas E. Rosenau, *A Celebration of Sex* (Nashville: Nelson, 1994), 86.

2. Bill Hull, *Anxious for Nothing* (Old Tappan, N. J.: Revell, 1987), 137-8.

3. John C. Maxwell, *Your Attitude, Key to Success* (San Bernardino, Calif.: Here's Life, 1984), 128.

4. Bill Hull, *Right Thinking* (Colorado Springs: NavPress, 1985), 68.

5. My thanks to author and speaker Cynthia Heald for this powerful comment that has so influenced my life (Lorraine).

6. Allender and Longman, *Intimate Allies*, 254.

7. Rosenau, *A Celebration of Sex*, 85.

8. Chart adapted from Maxwell, *Your Attitude, Key to Success*, 129.

Chapter 4: How Can I Relate When He's a Microwave and I'm a Crockpot?

1. James C. Dobson, "Dr. Dobson Answers Your Questions," *Colorado Springs Gazette Telegraph*, 11 September 1994, E3, quoting from Dr. Paul Popenoe, *Are Women Really Different?*

2. Donald Joy, "Innate Differences Between Men and Women," interview by James C. Dobson (Colorado Springs: Focus on the Family), tape CSO99/880.

3. Donna Jackson, "New News Relationship," *New Woman*, May 1998, 20.

4. Leslie Bennetts, "What Men Really Want," *Ladies Home Journal*, January 1996, 44.

5. Lesley Dorman, "The Three Styles of Sex," *Redbook*, March 1998, 93.

6. Dorman, "The Three Styles of Sex," 93.

7. John Gray, *Mars and Venus in the Bedroom* (New York: HarperCollins, 1995), 63.

8. Carolyn Hagan, "How to Make a Good 'O' Great," *Glamour*, May 1998, 287.

9. Hagan, "How to Make a Good 'O' Great," 285.

10. Hagan, "How to Make a Good 'O' Great," 284.

11. Gray, *Mars and Venus in the Bedroom*, 28.

12. Dennis Rainey, *Lonely Husbands, Lonely Wives* (Dallas: Word, 1989), 255. Used by permission.

Chapter 5: What Do I Do When I Don't Want to Do It?

1. Jane Brody, "Do You Need the Hormone of Desire?" *Readers Digest*, July 1998, 115.

2. Chris Bohjalian, "16 Natural Aphrodisiacs," *New Woman*, March 1998, 92.

3. Bel Henderson, "No One Is in the Mood All of the Time," *New Woman*, May 1998, 100.

Chapter 6: Where Can I Go to Buy a New Body?

1. "Mission Impossible," *People Weekly*, 3 June 1996, 73.

2. Alanna Nash, "Marvelous Meg," *Good Housekeeping*, July 1998, 99.

3. "Mission Impossible," 73.

4. Elizabeth Austin, "The Pound-a-Year Problem," *Self*, January 1998, 109-11.

5. "Snapshots" *USA Today*, 9 June 1998, sec. D, 1.

6. Austin, "The Pound-a-Year Problem," 109-11.

7. "Snapshots," 1.

8. Nancy Wartik, *Glamour*, May 1996, 223.

9. Gray, *Mars and Venus in the Bedroom,* 60.

10. Andrew M. Greeley, *Sexual Intimacy* (New York: Seabury Press, 1973), 86.

11. Lisa Douglass, "Orgasms: The Science," *New Woman,* June 1998, 126.

12. Charles R. Swindoll, *Growing Strong in the Seasons of Life* (Portland, Ore.: Multnomah, 1983), 271-2.

13. Alisa Bauman and Sari Harrar, *Fat to Firm* (Emmaus, Pa.: Rodale Press, Inc, 1998), 10.

14. Weigh Down Workshops/Seminars; P.O. Box 689099; Franklin, TN, 37068. Phone: (800) 844-5208. E-mail: info@wdworkshop.com

15. "Relationship News," *New Woman,* June 1997, 77.

16. Wartik, *Glamour,* 225.

17. Wartik, *Glamour,* 225.

18. "Sex and Your Health," *Colorado Springs Gazette,* 15 March 1998, Parade sec., 20.

19. "Sex and Your Health," 20.

20. "Sex and Your Health," 20.

Chapter 7: How Do I Make Love with Children Wrapped Around My Knees?

1. Mary Benin, quoted in Carol McD. Wallace, "7 Ways to Find Romance When You Have Little Kids," *Redbook,* July 1998, 96.

2. Jay Belsky and John Kelly, *The Transition to Parenthood,* quoted in Wallace, "7 Ways to Find Romance," 96.

3. Paul Pearsall, *Super Marital Sex* (New York: Ivy Books, 1987), 9.

4. Gary Chapman, *The Five Love Languages* (Chicago: Northfield Publishing, 1992), 156.

5. Lorraine Pintus, *Diapers, Pacifiers, and Other Holy Things* (Colorado Springs: Chariot Victor Publishing, 1995), 19-20.

Chapter 8: How Can I Get over the Guilt of Past Sexual Sin?

1. This prayer is modified from material taken from John Sandford and Paula Sandford, *The Transformation of the Inner Man* (Tulsa, Okla.: Victory House Inc., 1982), 269-94.

Chapter 9: I'm Attracted to Another Man! Help?

1. Ronnie Floyd, *The Power of Prayer and Fasting* (Nashville: Broadman, 1997), 13.

2. Charles Mylander, *Running the Red Lights: Putting the Brakes on Sexual Temptation* (Ventura, Calif.: Regal, 1986), 22.

Chapter 10: How Can I Remain Faithful in a Faithless World?

1. Stephen Strang, "Just Say No to Divorce," *Charisma,* May 1994, 108.

2. Ann Landers, *Colorado Springs Gazette,* 30 September 1996, Lifestyle sec., 3.

3. Lewis B. Smedes, *Sex for Christians* (Grand Rapids, Mich.: Eerdmans, 1976, 1994), 146-7.

4. James Dobson, *Colorado Springs Gazette,* 8 March 1998, Lifestyle sec., 3.

5. Natalie Gittelson, "Infidelity—Can You Forgive and Forget?" *Redbook,* November 1978, 192.

6. James C. Dobson, *Love Must be Tough* (Waco, Tex.: Word, 1983), 8.

Chapter 11: What Do I Do When HE Has a Headache?

1. Janet Wolfe, *What to Do When He Has a Headache* (New York: Hyperion, 1992), 2.

2. Dagmar O'Connor, *How to Make Love to the Same Person for the Rest of Your Life* (New York: Bantam Books, 1985), 293.

3. Wolfe, *What to Do,* 5-8.

4. C. H. Spurgeon, *Psalms 111-150,* vol. 3 of *The Treasury of David* (Grand Rapids, Mich.: Zondervan, 1966), 290.

5. Frank W. Cawood and Associates, *Natural Medicines and Cures Your Doctor Never Tells You About* (Peachtree City, Ga.: FC&A Publishing, 1997), 257.

6. *Physicians' Desk Reference* (Montvale, N. J.: Medical Economics Data Production Co., 1994). *PDR Guide to Drug Interactions Side Effect Indications* (Montvale, N. J.: Medical Economics Data Production Co., 1994), quoted in Cawood, *Natural Medicines and Cures,* 258.

7. Onan's brother died, and according to custom Onan was expected to impregnate his sister-in-law so she could have children to carry on his brother's name. Onan apparently wanted the inheritance for himself and his own children, so he practiced the withdrawal method of birth control: "But Onan knew that the offspring would not be his; so whenever he lay with his brother's wife, he spilled his semen on the ground to keep from producing offspring for his brother" (Genesis 38:9, NIV). Onan's sin was not masturbation but disobedience to God. See Rosenau, *A Celebration of Sex,* 151.

8. Rosenau, *A Celebration of Sex,* 152-3.

9. Clifford Penner and Joyce Penner, *The Gift of Sex* (Waco, Tex.: Word, 1981), 234.

10. *USA Today,* 31 March 1998, sec. D, 1-2.

11. According to the Food and Drug Administration, about "130 Americans who took the popular pill have died—most from heart attacks—since Viagra hit the market last spring." "Drug's Label Gets Additional Warning," *USA Today,* 25 November 1998, 5A.

12. Editors of Prevention Magazine Health Books, *How to Romance the Man You Love* (Emmaus, Pa.: Rodale Press, Inc., 1997), 14.

13. Editors of Prevention Magazine Health Books, *How to Romance the Man,* 15.

14. Chris Bohjalian, "16 Natural Aphrodisiacs," *New Woman,* March 1998, 16.

Chapter 12: How Can I Get Rid of Guilt over My Abortion?

1. Alan Guttmacher Institute, Special Research Affiliate of Planned Parenthood Federation of America, yearly abortion statistic.

2. Teri Reisser and Paul Reisser, *Identifying and Overcoming Post-Abortion Syndrome* (Colorado Springs: Focus on the Family, 1992), 17.

3. Written by a post-abortion woman and dedicated to her unborn child. This poem was sent anonymously to the Colorado Springs Pregnancy Center, Colorado Springs, Colorado, over ten years ago. We were unsuccessful in locating the author so we could credit her, but we pray she will be blessed by the knowledge that even today her words are encouraging mothers.

4. Anonymous, "What They Didn't Tell Me About Abortions," *Today's Christian Woman*, September–October 1996, 75.

5. Anonymous, "What They Didn't Tell Me," 76.

6. Reisser and Reisser, *Identifying and Overcoming Post-Abortion Syndrome*, 7.

7. Reisser and Reisser, *Identifying and Overcoming Post-Abortion Syndrome*, 9.

Chapter 13: My Husband Is into Pornography—What Should I Do?

1. Neal Clement, interview by Laurie Hall, *An Affair of the Mind* (Colorado Springs: Focus on the Family Publishing, 1996), 206.

2. Rosaline Bush, "Caught in a Raging River," *Family Voice*, May 1998, 15.

3. Hall, *An Affair of the Mind*, 207.

4. Hall, *An Affair of the Mind*, 11.

5. Hall, *An Affair of the Mind*, 12.

6. "Business of Pornography," *U.S. News and World Report*, 10 February 1997, 42-50.

7. Tom Helnen, "Sex on the Net," *Colorado Springs Gazette* 16 September 1997, LIF6.

8. Vic Sussman, "Sex on the Net," *USA Today*, 20 August 1997.

9. Debra Evans, *The Christian Woman's Guide to Sexuality* (Wheaton, Ill.: Crossway, 1997), 262.

10. Hall, *An Affair of the Mind*, 196.

11. Harry W. Schaumburg, *False Intimacy: Understanding the Struggle of Sexual Addiction* (Colorado Springs: NavPress, 1992), 20.

12. Tom Minnery, *Pornography: A Human Tragedy* (Wheaton, Ill.: Tyndale, 1987), 39.

13. Hall, *An Affair of the Mind*, 66.

14. Hall, *An Affair of the Mind*, 68.

15. Ron Miller, *Personality Traits of the Carnal Mind* (Hyde Park, Vt.: Entrust Media for Freedom Ministries, n.d.), 53.

16. Richard Foster, *Celebration of Discipline* (San Francisco: HarperCollins, 1978), 43-4.

17. Evans, *The Christian Woman's Guide to Sexuality*, 262.

18. Henry Cloud and John Townsend, *Boundaries* (Grand Rapids, Mich.: Zondervan, 1992), 31-2.

19. Several thoughts on this list were taken from Hall's book *An Affair of the Mind*. The majority of the list is summarized from a taped interview by the American Association of Counselors with Gene McDonnell. To obtain a copy of this tape, call 1-800-526-8673.

20. Schaumburg, *False Intimacy*, 23.

21. "Family Mail," *Focus on the Family Magazine,* July 1998, 16.

22. Lou Gonzales, *Colorado Springs Gazette*, 30 January 1998, Business sec., 6.

Chapter 14: Is It Possible to Get Beyond the Pain of Sexual Abuse?

1. Dan Allender, *The Wounded Heart* (Colorado Springs: NavPress, 1990), 41.

2. Marilyn Van Derbur Atler, interview in the *Colorado Springs Gazette.* 17 June 1998, A1, A12.

3. Atler, interview in the *Colorado Springs Gazette,* A12

Chapter 15: How Can Sex Go from Boring to Sizzling?

1. Paul Lee Tan, *Encyclopedia of 7700 Illustrations* (Rockville, Md.: Assurance Publishers, 1979), 215.

2. Mayo, *A Christian Guide to Sexual Counseling,* 70.

3. Franz Delitzsch, *Commentary on the Song of Songs and Ecclesiastes* (Grand Rapids: Eerdmans, n.d.), 45.

4. Harris H. Hirschberg, *Vestus Testamentum,* no. 4 (September 1961): 380. See also Delitzsch, *Commentary on the Song of Songs*, 88, where he equates the "garden" with the "woman chamber," i.e., vagina.

5. Joseph C. Dillow, *Solomon on Sex* (Nashville: Nelson, 1977), 132-4.

6. Delitzsch, *Commentary on the Song of Songs*, 122.

7. Dillow, *Solomon on Sex,* 134.

8. Stephen Covey, *The 7 Habits of Highly Successful People* (New York: Simon & Schuster, 1989), 98-9.

Chapter 16: What's the Big Deal About Orgasm?

1. Marjorie Ingall, "Romantic Getaways Gone Wrong: 7 True Tales," *Redbook*, August 1998, 66.

2. Douglass, "Orgasms: The Science," 109.

3. Marty Klein, "When Women Talk About Sex," *New Woman,* March 1997, 132.

4. Pearsall, *Super Marital Sex,* 123.

5. Rosenau, *A Celebration of Sex,* 47.

6. Rosenau, *A Celebration of Sex,* 54.

7. Catherine Dennis, "The Sex Skill You Can Practice Anywhere," *Redbook*, February 1997, 74.

8. Beverly Whipple, quoted in Dennis, "The Sex Skill," 76.

9. Dennis, "The Sex Skill," 76.

10. Linda DeVillers, quoted in Gail Hoch, "The Secrets of Highly Orgasmic Women," *Redbook*, November 1996, 101.

11. Gail Hoch, "The Secrets of Highly Orgasmic Women," 99.

12. Rosenau, *A Celebration of Sex,* 52.

13. Mary Ann Mayo and Joseph L. Mayo, *The Sexual Woman* (Eugene, Ore.: Harvest House, 1987), 33-4.

14. Ed Wheat and Gaye Wheat, *Intended for Pleasure* (Old Tappan, N. J.: Revell, 1977), 103-11.

15. Rosenau, *A Celebration of Sex,* 242. For further information, read chapter 18 in *A Celebration of Sex,* "Women Becoming More Easily Orgasmic," 241-54.

Chapter 17: What's Not Okay in Bed?

1. W. F. Arndt and F. W. Gingrich, *A Greek-English Lexicon of the New Testament* (Grand Rapids, Mich.: Zondervan, 1957), s.v. "molvno" (impure).

2. Bromley, *The International Standard Bible Encyclopedia,* s.v. "crime."

3. *The Lexicon Webster Dictionary,* vol. 2, s.v. "sodomy."

4. Bromley, *The International Standard Bible Encyclopedia,* s.v. "sodomite."

5. R. Laird Harris, Gleason Archer, Bruce Waltke, *Theological Wordbook of the Old Testament,* vol. 2 (Chicago: Moody, 1980), s.v. "gadesh."

6. Penner and Penner, *The Gift of Sex,* 228.

7. Dillow, *Solomon on Sex,* 31.

8. Rosenau, *A Celebrations of Sex,* 57.

9. Smedes, *Sex for Christians,* 211.

10. Wheat and Wheat, *Intended for Pleasure,* 76-7.

11. From *Legal Briefs* by Michael D. Shook & Jeffrey D. Meyer (New York: Macmillan, 1995) and from *Details,* June 1993, quoted in *Marie Claire,* November 1996, 78-9.

12. Smedes, *Sex for Christians,* 212.

Chapter 18: Are Quickies Okay with God?

1. Wheat and Wheat, *Intended for Pleasure,* 193.

2. Wolfe, *What to Do,* 22.

3. Karen S. Peterson, "Study finds highly educated have less sex," *USA Today,* 14 January 1998, 1A.

4. "Sex Sex Sex," *Jane Magazine,* March 1998, 70.

5. Mayo, *A Christian Guide to Sexual Counseling,* 82-3.

6. Mayo, *A Christian Guide to Sexual Counseling,* 83.

7. Evans, *The Christian Woman's Guide to Sexuality,* 130.

8. Smedes, *Sex for Christians,* 210.

9. Mayo, *A Christian Guide to Sexual Counseling,* 201.

10. Smedes, *Sex for Christians*, 211.

11. Wolfe, *What to Do,* 243.

12. Barbara DeAngelis, *Ask Barbara* (New York: Bantam, 1997), 169.

13. Gray, *Mars and Venus in the Bedroom,* 77.

14. Gray, *Mars and Venus in the Bedroom,* 139.

15. Gray, *Mars and Venus in the Bedroom,* 92.

Chapter 19: How Can I Recapture the Passion?

1. Ann Landers, *Colorado Springs Gazette,* 12 March 1998, Lifestyle sec., 6.

2. Pearsall, *Super Marital Sex,* 15-6.

3. Judith Newman, "How to Be a Sex Goddess in Your Own Home," *Redbook,* October 1996, 114.

4. Editors of *Prevention* Magazine Health Books, *How to Romance the Man,* 20.

5. Rick Bundschuh and Dave Gilbert, *Romance Rekindled* (Eugene, Ore.: Harvest House, 1988), 64.

6. Bundschuh and Gilbert, *Romance Rekindled,* 193.

7. Ann Landers, *Colorado Springs Gazette* 6 June 1998, Lifestyle sec., 5.

8. Editors of *Prevention* Magazine Health Books, *How to Romance the Man,* 3.

Scripture Index

Topical Index